Strength Training Past 50

Third Edition

Wayne L. Westcott

Thomas R. Baechle

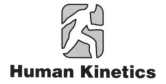

Human Kinetics

Library of Congress Cataloging-in-Publication Data

Westcott, Wayne L., 1949-
 Strength training past 50 / Wayne L. Westcott, Thomas R. Baechle. -- Third edition.
    pages cm
 Includes bibliographical references.
 1. Weight training. 2. Physical fitness for middle-aged persons. I. Baechle, Thomas R., 1943- II. Title. III.
Title: Strength training past fifty.
 GV546.W47 2015
 613.7'130844--dc23

                              2014045517

ISBN: 978-1-4504-9791-6 (print)

The web addresses cited in this text were current as of January 2015, unless otherwise noted.

Acquisitions Editor: Justin Klug; **Senior Managing Editor:** Amy Stahl; **Associate Managing Editor:** Nicole Moore; **Copyeditor**: Jan Feeney; **Permissions Manager:** Martha Gullo; **Graphic Designer:** Human Kinetics staff; **Cover Designer:** Keith Blomberg; **Photograph (cover):** Jason Allen; **Photographs (interior):** Neil Bernstein; **Visual Production Assistant:** Joyce Brumfield; **Photo Production Manager:** Jason Allen; **Art Manager:** Kelly Hendren; **Associate Art Manager:** Alan L. Wilborn; **Illustrations:** © Human Kinetics, unless otherwise noted; **Printer:** Versa Press

We thank The Refinery in Champaign, Illinois, for assistance in providing a location for the photo shoot for this book.

Printed in the United States of America   10 9 8 7 6 5 4 3 2 1

The paper in this book is certified under a sustainable forestry program.

Human Kinetics
Website: www.HumanKinetics.com

United States: Human Kinetics
P.O. Box 5076
Champaign, IL 61825-5076
800-747-4457
e-mail: humank@hkusa.com

Canada: Human Kinetics
475 Devonshire Road Unit 100
Windsor, ON N8Y 2L5
800-465-7301 (in Canada only)
e-mail: info@hkcanada.com

Europe: Human Kinetics
107 Bradford Road
Stanningley
Leeds LS28 6AT, United Kingdom
+44 (0) 113 255 5665
e-mail: hk@hkeurope.com

Australia: Human Kinetics
57A Price Avenue
Lower Mitcham, South Australia 5062
08 8372 0999
e-mail: info@hkaustralia.com

New Zealand: Human Kinetics
P.O. Box 80
Torrens Park, South Australia 5062
0800 222 062
e-mail: info@hknewzealand.com

E6328

Strength Training Past 50

Third Edition

Contents

Exercise Finder

MACHINE EXERCISES				
Exercises	Primary muscles worked	Other muscles worked	Single-joint or multijoint	Page #
Leg exercises				
Leg extension	Quadriceps		Single-joint	60
Leg curl	Hamstrings		Single-joint	61
Leg press	Quadriceps, hamstrings, gluteals	Hip adductors, gastrocnemius, soleus	Multijoint	62
Hip adduction	Hip adductors		Single-joint	64
Hip abduction	Hip abductors		Single-joint	65
Heel raise	Gastrocnemius, soleus		Single-joint	66
Core exercises				
Low back extension	Erector spine		Single-joint	67
Abdominal flexion	Rectus abdominis		Single-joint	68
Rotary torso	Rectus abdominis, external obliques, internal obliques		Single-joint	69
Chest exercises				
Chest crossover	Pectoralis major, anterior deltoids		Single-joint	70
Chest press	Pectoralis major, anterior deltoids, triceps	Serratus anterior	Multijoint	71
Incline press	Pectoralis major, anterior deltoids, triceps	Serratus anterior, upper trapezius	Multijoint	72
Shoulder exercises				
Lateral raise	Deltoids	Upper trapezius	Single-joint	73
Shoulder press	Deltoids, triceps, upper trapezius		Multijoint	74
Upper-back exercises				
Pullover	Latissimus dorsi	Triceps, posterior deltoids, teres major	Single-joint	76
Lat pulldown	Latissimus dorsi, biceps	Posterior deltoids, rhomboids, middle trapezius, teres major	Multijoint	78
Seated row	Latissimus dorsi, biceps	Posterior deltoids, rhomboids, middle trapezius, teres major	Multijoint	79
Weight-assisted chin-up	Latissimus dorsi, biceps	Posterior deltoids, rhomboids, middle trapezius, teres major	Multijoint	80
Rowing	Latissimus dorsi, biceps, posterior deltoids, rhomboids, middle trapezius	Teres major	Multijoint	82
Chest and back-of-arm exercise				
Weight-assisted bar dip	Pectoralis major, triceps	Anterior deltoids, latissimus dorsi, teres major, pectoralis minor	Multijoint	83

MACHINE EXERCISES *(continued)*				
Exercises	Primary muscles worked	Other muscles worked	Single-joint or multijoint	Page #
Arm exercises				
Biceps curl	Biceps	Wrist flexors	Single-joint	84
Triceps extension	Triceps		Single-joint	85
Triceps press	Triceps, pectoralis major, anterior deltoids	Pectoralis minor	Multijoint	86
Triceps press-down	Triceps	Pectoralis major, latissimus dorsi, rectus abdominis	Single-joint	87
Neck exercises				
Neck extension	Neck extensors		Single-joint	88
Neck flexion	Neck flexors		Single-joint	89
FREE-WEIGHT EXERCISES (KETTLEBELLS, DUMBBELLS, BARBELL)				
Exercises	Primary muscles worked	Other muscles worked	Single-joint or multijoint	Page #
Leg exercises				
Squat: kettlebells or dumbbells	Quadriceps, hamstrings, gluteals	Erector spinae	Multijoint	92
Squat: barbell	Quadriceps, hamstrings, gluteals	Erector spinae	Multijoint	94
Step-up: kettlebells or dumbbells	Quadriceps, hamstrings, gluteals	Erector spinae	Multijoint	96
Lunge: kettlebells or dumbbells	Quadriceps, hamstrings, gluteals	Erector spinae	Multijoint	97
Heel raise: kettlebells or dumbbells	Gastrocnemius, soleus		Single-joint	98
Heel raise: barbell	Gastrocnemius, soleus		Single-joint	100
Front squat: dumbbell	Gluteus maximus, hamstrings, quadriceps		Multijoint	102
Swing: kettlebell	Gluteus maximus, hamstrings, quadriceps, deltoids		Multijoint	104
Core exercises				
Side bend: kettlebell or dumbbell	Rectus abdominis, external obliques, internal obliques		Single-joint	106
Deadlift: kettlebells or dumbbells	Erector spinae, quadriceps, hamstrings, gluteals		Multijoint	107
Deadlift: barbell	Erector spinae, quadriceps, hamstrings, gluteals		Multi-joint	108
Chest exercises				
Chest fly: dumbbells	Pectoralis major, anterior deltoids	Serratus anterior	Single-joint	109
Bench press: dumbbells	Pectoralis major, anterior deltoids, triceps	Serratus anterior	Multijoint	110
Bench press: barbell	Pectoralis major, anterior deltoids, triceps	Serratus anterior	Multijoint	112

FREE-WEIGHT EXERCISES (KETTLEBELLS, DUMBBELLS, BARBELL)　*(continued)*				
Exercises	Primary muscles worked	Other muscles worked	Single-joint or multijoint	Page #
Chest and shoulder exercises				
Incline press: barbell	Pectoralis major, anterior deltoids, triceps	Serratus anterior	Multijoint	114
Incline press: dumbbells	Pectoralis major, anterior deltoids, triceps	Serratus anterior	Multijoint	116
Shoulder exercises				
Lateral raise: dumbbells	Deltoids		Single-joint	118
Seated press: dumbbells	Deltoids, triceps, upper trapezius		Multijoint	119
Alternating shoulder press: dumbbells	Deltoids, triceps, upper trapezius		Multijoint	120
Standing press: barbell	Deltoids, triceps, upper trapezius		Multijoint	122
Upper-back exercises				
Pullover: dumbbell	Latissimus dorsi	Triceps	Single-joint	124
One-arm row: kettlebell or dumbbell	Latissimus dorsi, biceps	Posterior deltoid, rhomboid, middle trapezius, teres major	Multijoint	126
Double bent-over row: kettlebells or dumbbells	Latissimus dorsi, rhomboids	Posterior deltoid, biceps, middle trapezius, teres minor	Multijoint	128
Reverse fly: dumbbells	Latissimus dorsi, upper trapezius, rhomboids	Triceps	Single-joint	129
Front-of-arm exercises				
Standing biceps curl: barbell	Biceps	Wrist flexors, latissimus dorsi, pectoralis major	Single-joint	130
Standing biceps curl: dumbbells	Biceps	Wrist flexors latissimus dorsi, pectoralis major	Single-joint	131
Incline curl: dumbbells	Biceps	Wrist flexors, latissimus dorsi, pectoralis major	Single-joint	132
Preacher curl: dumbbells	Biceps		Single-joint	133
Concentration curl: dumbbell	Biceps		Single-joint	134
Back-of-arm exercises				
Overhead triceps extension: dumbbell	Triceps	Deltoids	Single-joint	135
Lying triceps extension: dumbbells	Triceps	Deltoids	Single-joint	136
Triceps kickback: dumbbell	Triceps	Deltoids	Single-joint	138
Neck exercises				
Shrug: barbell	Upper trapezius		Single-joint	140
Shrug: dumbbells or kettlebells	Upper trapezius		Single-joint	141

ALTERNATIVE-EQUIPMENT EXERCISES

Exercises	Primary muscles worked	Other muscles worked	Single-joint or multijoint	Page #
Leg exercises				
Wall squat: exercise ball with dumbbells	Quadriceps, hamstrings, gluteals	Erector spinae	Multijoint	144
Heel pull: exercise ball	Hamstrings, hip flexors	Rectus abdominis, rectus femoris	Multijoint	145
Leg lift: exercise ball	Quadriceps, hip flexors, rectus abdominis	Hip adductors	Single-joint	146
Squat: resistance band	Gluteus maximus, hamstrings, quadriceps	Erector spinae	Multijoint	148
Core exercises				
Trunk extension: body weight	Erector spinae		Single-joint	150
Trunk extension: exercise ball	Erector spinae		Single-joint	151
Twisting trunk curl: body weight	Rectus abdominis, rectus femoris, hip flexors, external obliques, internal obliques		Multijoint	152
Trunk curl: exercise ball	Rectus abdominis		Single-joint	154
Side plank: body weight	Rectus abdominis	External obliques, internal obliques, erector spinae, pectoralis major, anterior deltoids, triceps	Single-joint	156
Sit-up: body weight	Rectus abdominis	Rectus femoris, hip flexors	Multijoint	158
Chest exercises				
Chest press: resistance band	Pectoralis major, triceps, anterior deltoids	Serratus anterior	Multijoint	159
Push-up: exercise ball	Pectoralis major, anterior deltoids, triceps, rectus abdominis	Serratus anterior	Multijoint	160
Bar dip: body weight	Pectoralis major, anterior deltoids, triceps	Latissimus dorsi, teres major, pectoralis minor	Multijoint	161
Shoulder exercises				
Lateral raise: resistance band	Deltoids	Upper trapezius	Single-joint	162
Seated press: resistance band	Deltoids, triceps	Upper trapezius	Multijoint	164
Upper-back exercises				
Chin-up: body weight	Latissimus dorsi, biceps	Posterior deltoids, rhomboids, middle trapezius, teres major	Multijoint	166
Upright row: resistance band	Deltoids, upper trapezius	Biceps	Multijoint	167
Seated row: resistance band	Latissimus dorsi, biceps	Posterior deltoids, rhomboids, middle trapezius, teres major	Multijoint	168
Arm exercises				
Biceps curl: resistance band	Biceps	Wrist flexors, pectoralis major, latissimus dorsi	Single-joint	170
Bench dip: exercise ball	Triceps, pectoralis major, anterior deltoids	Latissimus dorsi, teres major, pectoralis minor	Multijoint	171
One-arm triceps extension: resistance band	Triceps	Deltoids, upper trapezius	Single-joint	172
Walk-out: exercise ball	Triceps, pectoralis major, anterior deltoids	Rectus abdominis	Multijoint	174
Neck exercise				
Shrug: resistance band	Upper trapezius	Wrist flexors	Single-joint	175

Acknowledgments

We are most appreciative for the privilege of publishing the third edition of *Strength Training Past 50*, and we express our sincere thanks to our excellent Human Kinetics editorial team of Amy Stahl, Justin Klug, Jan Feeney, and Roger Earle. Thanks also to our outstanding photographer Neil Bernstein and exemplary exercise models, Keith Blomberg, Tim Ellis, Greg Edwards, Dar Bouck, Joella Evans, and Dick Raymond. We are grateful to our institutions for their support of our research studies, publications, and presentations as well as to our professional colleague Rita LaRosa Loud for her expert assistance with our chapter manuscripts and for being an exercise model. We are most thankful for the friendship we share with each other; for the love, patience, and prayers of our wives, Claudia Westcott and Susan Baechle; and for God's enabling grace in writing this book.

Introduction

Welcome to one of the most exciting and beneficial activities that you can do at any age, especially after age 50. While strength training is effective for increasing strength, size, and function for all age groups, performing regular resistance exercise is particularly important for older adults. This is because men and women over the age of 50 typically lose 5 to 10 pounds of muscle tissue every decade unless they engage in resistance training. Muscle loss has major health implications because it is associated with bone loss, physical dysfunction, metabolic slowdown, and fat gain. Fortunately, sensible strength training can reverse these degenerative processes and reduce the risk of related health issues such as osteoporosis, obesity, diabetes, heart disease, low back pain, arthritis, fibromyalgia, and psychological problems.

Chapter 1 presents a wealth of research-based information on the health benefits that can result from regular resistance exercise. You may be surprised to learn about the many physiological adaptations that are associated with strength training and how these are especially applicable to those over age 50. Assuming that you would like to attain more muscular fitness, greater functional abilities, better health, and higher quality of life, you should be eager to read chapter 2, which presents the steps that enable you to start your strength training program.

The next chapter sets the foundation for successful and sustainable strength training experiences. Chapter 3 describes the research-based recommendations for performing resistance exercise in a safe manner with respect to training exercises, frequency, resistance, repetitions, sets, progression, and related workout factors.

Chapter 4 presents information on selecting and using strength training equipment, including resistance machines, free weights, resistance bands, kettlebells, and stability balls. This is a nuts-and-bolts chapter that prepares you to select the most appropriate resistance equipment for the exercises in chapters 6, 7, and 8.

Chapter 5 discusses the basic exercise techniques for performing strength training properly and productively. This chapter includes information on correct grips, standard stances, movement paths, exercise speeds, breathing patterns, and other factors of exercise performance.

The key to safe, successful, and sustainable strength training programs is proper execution of the resistance exercises. Chapter 6 contains instructions and photos on performing machine exercises. Chapter 7 details execution of barbell, dumbbell, and kettlebell exercises along with photos of the beginning and ending positions for these free-weight exercises. Chapter 8 presents performance guidelines for alternative resistance training modes, including body-weight exercises, resistance band exercises, and stability ball training.

Once you know how to perform resistance exercises safely and effectively, you need to select the most appropriate strength training program to accommodate your present level of physical ability and to achieve your health and fitness objectives.

Chapter 9 presents basic strength training workouts for machines, free weights, and alternative equipment (body weight, exercise balls, and resistance bands). For each equipment category we provide two training programs, a brief workout and a standard routine, both of which should enable you to attain excellent results in your available time frame. Chapter 10 presents advanced strength training workouts for machines, free weights, and alternative equipment (body weight, exercise balls, and resistance bands). For each category, we provide a high-load training protocol and a high-intensity training protocol. These advanced resistance exercise programs should enable you to attain relatively high levels of muscular strength in a sensible and systematic manner.

If you are a sport enthusiast, you may want to progress to a more specialized strength training program. Chapter 11 presents resistance exercises and training protocols for the popular athletic activities of running, cycling, swimming, skiing, tennis, and golf. For each sport, we provide training programs using machine exercises, free-weight exercises, and body-weight and resistance band exercises.

Research has demonstrated the importance of proper nutrition for enhancing resistance training results, especially with respect to muscle development and bone density. In addition to presenting principles of healthy eating and dietary recommendations, chapter 12 discusses the latest research on obtaining optimal protein intake for musculoskeletal health and fitness in over-50 exercisers.

Congratulations on your decision to make an important change in lifestyle—that is, performing regular resistance exercise. Comparatively speaking, the time commitment is low and the health and fitness benefits are high. Without question, the third edition of *Strength Training Past 50* provides the information you need for safe and efficient resistance exercise that will help you to look, feel, and function better throughout your life. Just make sure that you have your physician's approval and that you adhere to the research-based recommendations presented in the following pages.

Key to Muscles

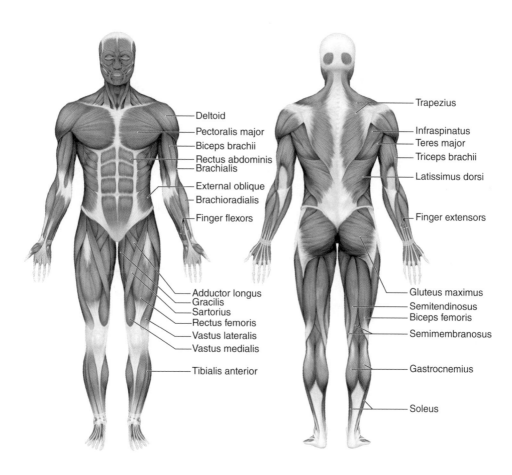

Deltoid

Pectoralis major

Biceps brachii

Rectus abdominis

Brachialis

External oblique

Brachioradialis

Finger flexors

Adductor longus

Gracilis

Sartorius

Rectus femoris

Vastus lateralis

Vastus medialis

Tibialis anterior

Trapezius

Infraspinatus

Teres major

Triceps brachii

Latissimus dorsi

Finger extensors

Gluteus maximus

Semitendinosus

Biceps femoris

Semimembranosus

Gastrocnemius

Soleus

Benefits of Strength Training

We live in a society characterized by too little physical activity and too many passive pursuits. The predictable result of our inactive lifestyle is an almost unavoidable increase in body weight. Indeed, as assessed by body mass index (BMI), more than 65 percent of American adults may be classified as overweight or obese (Hedley et al. 2004). However, because BMI calculations do not account for the components of lean (muscle) weight and fat weight, these ratings significantly underestimate the percentage of American adults who have unhealthy amounts of body fat. In fact, approximately 80 percent of men and women in their 50s and older have too little muscle and too much fat (Flegal et al. 2010).

Research indicates that there is a critical cause-and-effect relationship between muscle loss and fat gain. Unless you perform some type of muscle strengthening activity, you will lose about 5 pounds (2.3 kg) of lean (muscle) weight every decade of adult life (Frontera et al. 2000). Because muscle tissue is metabolically active 24 hours a day, the 5-pound-per-decade decrease in muscle mass typically results in a reduction in resting metabolic rate of 3 percent per decade (Keys et al. 1973). A lower resting metabolic rate means that fewer calories are burned on a daily basis; therefore, more calories are stored as body fat. Because resting metabolism accounts for approximately 70 percent of the calories used every day, metabolic slowdown is a major factor in fat gain during aging (Wolfe 2006).

Due largely to the reduction in resting metabolic rate, the 5-pound-per-decade muscle loss is accompanied by a 15-pound-per-decade (~7 kg) fat gain. Mathematically, this represents a 10-pound-per-decade (4.6 kg) increase in body weight. However, when you look at the real impact of 5 pounds less muscle and 15 pounds more fat, you actually experience a 20-pound (~9 kg) undesirable change in body composition. If you fast-forward from age 20 to age 50, the scale may show a 30-pound (13.6 kg) increase in body weight. However, over these 3 decades the average 50-year-old has lost about 15 pounds of muscle and added about 45 pounds (20.4) of fat, for a 60-pound reversal in body composition.

Unfortunately, this major change in body composition adversely affects personal health as well as physical fitness. Problems associated with muscle loss and fat gain include obesity, osteoporosis, diabetes, high blood pressure, high blood cholesterol, heart disease, stroke, arthritis, low back pain, and many types of cancer, as well as all-cause mortality.

Fortunately, muscle loss is reversible, and research reveals that resistance exercise is highly effective for increasing muscle mass at all ages (Campbell et al. 1994;

Fiatarone et al. 1990; Westcott et al. 2009). Maintaining a strong muscular system is so important that a leading medical research journal (*American College of Sports Medicine's Current Sports Medicine Reports*) advocates a public health mandate for sensible strength training (Phillips and Winett 2010). Indeed, because the rate of muscle loss nearly doubles after the fifth decade of life, it is essential for men and women over age 50 to engage in regular resistance exercise.

REBUILDING MUSCLE

Dozens of studies have demonstrated that a relatively brief program of resistance exercise (20 to 40 minutes per session, 2 or 3 days per week) can rebuild muscle tissue in people between 50 and 90 years of age. Most of these research programs have resulted in 3 to 4 pounds more muscle after just 3 to 4 months of strength training (Campbell et al. 1994; Pratley et al. 1994). We completed a large study to determine the effects of resistance exercise on body composition and blood pressure in which the major focus was on muscle rebuilding. More than 1,600 study participants (average age of 54 years) performed 10 weeks of carefully supervised resistance exercise. Their strength training program required just 1 set of 12 standard resistance machine exercises, 2 or 3 days per week, using a weight load that could be performed 8 to 12 repetitions. Whenever participants completed 12 repetitions with proper technique, the weight load was increased by approximately 5 percent. After 10 weeks of regular training with this basic and brief exercise protocol, the participants averaged a 3-pound increase in lean (muscle) weight. We also found that both training frequencies (2 days/week and 3 days/week) produced the same lean weight gain, and there were no significant differences in the rate of muscle development among the younger, middle-aged, and older adult age groups (Westcott et al. 2009).

RECHARGING METABOLISM

Resistance training has a dual impact on metabolic rate because it increases energy use during both the exercise session and during the muscle recovery and rebuilding period (up to 3 days after each workout). Because resistance training is a vigorous activity, relatively high levels of energy production are required for performing the exercises. For example, during a circuit strength training program, you are likely to burn 8 to 10 calories per minute, or 160 to 200 calories over a 20-minute exercise session. Because of the high-intensity aspect of resistance exercise, you are also likely to burn 25 percent more calories during the hour after a circuit strength training session. So the same 20-minute circuit strength training session is actually responsible for burning 200 to 250 calories in an 80-minute time frame. However, there's even better news. Research has shown that exercisers have a 5 percent increase in resting energy expenditure for 72 hours after resistance training sessions (Hackney et al. 2008; Heden at al. 2011). In a classic study, both a 15-minute strength workout (10 exercises × 1 set each) and 35-minute strength workout (10 exercises × 3 sets each) increased the trainees' resting energy expenditure by 5 percent (approximately 100 calories per day) for 3 full days after the exercise session (Heden at al. 2011). This large elevation in resting metabolic rate is due to the muscle microtrauma caused by resistance exercise and the resulting muscle remodeling processes that require relatively large amounts of energy for protein synthesis and tissue building. This is why every pound of skeletal muscle in untrained individuals uses about 6 calories every day at rest compared to that of strength-trained individuals whose muscles use about 9 calories per pound every day at rest, for a 50 percent higher muscle metabolism.

Many other studies have demonstrated even greater increases in resting metabolic rate (7 to 8 percent) after about 3 months of standard strength training (Broeder et al. 1992; Campbell et al. 1994; Pratley et al. 1994). The higher daily energy use is due to the development of new muscle tissue. At a daily energy cost of 9 calories per pound, 3 pounds more muscle increases resting metabolic rate by almost 30 additional calories every day. The more muscle you develop through regular resistance exercise, the more calories you use daily for tissue repair, remodeling, and rebuilding processes, and this is reflected in a significantly higher resting metabolism. Remember that resting metabolism accounts for up to 70 percent of daily calorie burn, so a higher resting metabolic rate is very beneficial for fat loss and weight management.

REDUCING FAT

Most people experience fat accumulation during aging, even if eating patterns remain essentially the same. As you are now aware, the loss of muscle and the resulting reduction in resting metabolism account for much of the fat gain. Excess fat detracts from physical appearance. As mentioned earlier, high levels of body fat also increase the risk of numerous health problems, including high blood pressure, high blood cholesterol, high blood sugar, diabetes, heart disease, stroke, arthritis, low back pain, and many types of cancer.

Fortunately, the same strength training studies that showed a 3- to 4-pound increase in lean (muscle) weight and a 7 to 8 percent increase in resting metabolic rate also demonstrated a 3- to 4-pound decrease in fat weight (Campbell et al. 1994; Pratley et al. 1994). Equally important, research reveals that resistance exercise is an effective means for reducing abdominal and intra-abdominal fat (especially in older men and women), which, among other benefits, reduces the risk of developing type 2 diabetes (Treuth et al. 1994; Treuth et al. 1995). When coupled with a modest decrease in daily food intake, 10 weeks of basic resistance exercise can result in a 6- to 9-pound fat loss. For example, in a study by Westcott and colleagues (2013), participants (average age 59 years) performed a standard strength training program and followed a moderate-calorie nutrition plan (1,200 to 1,500 calories/day for women and 1,500 to 1,800 calories/day for men). After 10 weeks, the older participants lost 9 pounds of fat weight and added 3 pounds of lean (muscle) weight for a 12-pound improvement in their body composition. They also reduced their resting blood pressure by almost 6 mmHg systolic and almost 4 mmHg diastolic, which is another excellent reason for combining a sensible strength training program and a sound nutrition program.

REDUCING RESTING BLOOD PRESSURE

Resting blood pressure plays a major role in cardiovascular health. Generally speaking, resting blood pressure should be approximately 120 mmHg during heart muscle contractions (known as systolic blood pressure) and approximately 80 mmHg between contractions (known as diastolic blood pressure). Unfortunately, approximately one-third of American adults have high blood pressure (hypertension), which is a major risk factor for cardiovascular disease (Ong et al. 2007). It is, therefore, encouraging to learn that numerous research studies have shown significant reductions in resting blood pressure readings after 2 or more months of standard or circuit-style strength training. Most of these studies have resulted in lower systolic and diastolic blood pressure readings, with an average systolic decrease of 6 mmHg and an average diastolic decrease of 5 mmHg. In our study of more than 1,600 men and women with an average age of 54 years, the relatively brief strength training program (1 set of 12 resistance machine exercises, 3 days/ week) reduced resting systolic blood pressure by more than 4 mmHg and diastolic blood pressure by more than 2 mmHg after just 10 weeks of training (Westcott et al. 2009). Although all exercise raises systolic resting blood pressure during the activity session, research indicates that sensible strength training produces elevations in exercise blood pressure similar to those seen with aerobic activities such as running and cycling. Consequently, unless your physician states otherwise, properly performed resistance exercise should be a safe physical activity that typically results in reduced resting blood pressure.

IMPROVING BLOOD LIPID PROFILES

Blood lipid profiles are standard medical measures of the fat that is transported through the cardiovascular system. These include HDL (good) cholesterol, LDL (bad) cholesterol, and triglycerides. Almost half of American adults have undesirable blood lipid levels, which increase the risk for heart disease (Lloyd-Jones et al. 2009). Fortunately, a large number of studies have shown positive effects of resistance exercise on blood lipid profiles. According to the American College of Sports Medicine (2009), research has revealed favorable increases of 8 to 21 percent in HDL (good) cholesterol, favorable decreases of 13 to 23 percent in LDL (bad) cholesterol, and favorable reductions of 11 to 18 percent in triglycerides resulting from regular strength training. Although genetic factors may influence the impact of resistance exercise on blood lipid levels, studies with older adults have been especially encouraging in this area. You can, therefore, feel confident that improved blood lipid profiles may be an important health benefit of strength training for adults of all ages.

ENHANCING POSTCORONARY PERFORMANCE

Many older adults have had cardiovascular health problems, including coronary artery disease, heart attack, and heart surgery. Research has revealed that these individuals can perform appropriate resistance exercise safely and effectively.

This is good news because strength training provides many health and fitness benefits to postcoronary patients. In addition to reducing resting blood pressure and improving blood lipid profiles, resistance exercise has proved to be a productive means for attaining and maintaining desirable body weight, increasing muscle mass and strength, improving physical performance, speeding the recovery from a cardiovascular event, and enhancing self-concept and self-efficacy in postcoronary patients (Faigenbaum et al. 1990; Marzolini et al. 2008; Stewart et al. 1988).

RESISTING DIABETES

The increasing number of overweight and obese adults is essentially paralleled by an increasing prevalence of type 2 diabetes. Unless current trends in these closely related health issues change for the better, it is predicted that by the year 2050 as many as 1 in 3 American adults will have type 2 diabetes (Boyle 2010). Fortunately, people who have desirable body weights and moderate to high levels of muscular fitness have a very low risk of developing type 2 diabetes. Because muscles function as the engines of the body and serve as sugar (glycogen) storehouses, many researchers have examined the effects of resistance exercise on factors associated with diabetes, such as insulin sensitivity and glycemic control. Almost all of these studies have shown significant improvements in insulin sensitivity and glycemic control after several weeks of strength training (Castaneda et al. 2002; Dunstan et al. 2002; Holten et al. 2004). As presented previously, resistance exercise also reduces abdominal and intra-abdominal fat, which appears to be particularly important for diabetes prevention. The diabetes-specific benefits provided by resistance exercise have led researchers to conclude that strength training should be recommended for both the prevention and management of type 2 diabetes (Flack et al. 2011). In fact, the American Diabetes Association exercise guidelines call for resistance training sessions that address all of the major muscle groups, 3 days per week, with each exercise performed for 1 to 3 sets of 8 to 10 repetitions at a high intensity (Standards of Medical Care in Diabetes 2006).

INCREASING BONE DENSITY

The National Osteoporosis Foundation (2009) states that approximately 35 million Americans have insufficient bone mass (osteopenia) and that another 10 million adults, 8 million of whom are women, have frail bones (osteoporosis). According to the U.S. Department of Health and Human Services (2004), osteoporosis will cause bone fractures in almost 1 of every 3 women and 1 of every 6 men. Although many factors influence bone thinning, it is clear that muscle loss is closely associated with bone loss. Research reveals that men and women who do not perform resistance exercise reduce their bone density by 1 to 3 percent every year of adult life, which represents a bone loss of 10 to 30 percent every decade.

Fortunately, strength training increases both muscle mass and bone mass. Numerous studies have shown significant increases in bone mineral density after several months of regular resistance exercise. Interestingly, the rate of improvement in bone mass resulting from strength training is 1 to 3 percent, which essentially reverses the bone loss that would otherwise be experienced by nonexercising adults. Although most of the strength training studies related to bone mass have been conducted with women, research with men has demonstrated even greater effects of resistance exercise, with increases in bone mineral density exceeding 3 percent (Almstedt et al. 2011).

Clearly, regular resistance training is the most productive means for developing a strong and injury-resistant musculoskeletal system. When looking specifically at osteoporosis prevention, research indicates that strength training has a more potent effect on bone density than other physical activities (aerobic and weight bearing), which renders resistance exercise an important lifestyle component for aging adults (Gutin and Kasper 1992).

DECREASING PHYSICAL DISCOMFORT

Research indicates that a large percentage of people with lower back pain can reduce discomfort by strengthening their low back muscles. Although not all low back pain is associated with weak muscles, several studies have shown significant relief in most of their participants after performing 8 to 24 weeks of specific low back resistance exercise (Hayden et al. 2005; Liddle et al. 2004; Risch et al. 1993). Strong low back muscles provide greater stability and support for spinal column structures as well as better shock absorption from landing forces such as running, jumping, and dancing.

Resistance exercise has also proven helpful for people who have arthritis and fibromyalgia. Although the mechanisms responsible for improvement of these maladies are not fully understood, research clearly demonstrates that strength training may result in reduced arthritic discomfort and pain associated with fibromyalgia (Focht 2006; Lange et al. 2008; Bircan et al. 2008).

ENHANCING MENTAL HEALTH

Mental health includes both psychological factors and cognitive abilities. Research has revealed significant improvements in depression, physical self-concept, fatigue, revitalization, tranquility, tension, positive engagement, and overall mood disturbance among adults and older adults (Annesi and Westcott 2004; Annesi and Westcott 2007). Depression may be particularly problematic for people over age 50 because it can seriously decrease functionality. It is, therefore, encouraging to learn the findings from a Harvard University study in which 80 percent of the participants were no longer clinically depressed after just 10 weeks of resistance exercise (Singh et al. 1997).

In addition to numerous studies showing favorable psychological outcomes from strength training, research has demonstrated significant cognitive benefits from resistance exercise (Busse et al. 2008; Cassilhas et al. 2007). Perhaps most prominent among these favorable findings is memory improvement in older adults.

REVITALIZING MUSCLE CELLS

Muscles function as the engines for the body, and mitochondria serve as the power sources of muscle cells. One undesirable aspect of the aging process is mitochondria deterioration in both content and function. Fortunately, studies have shown that circuit-style strength training, characterized by short rests between successive exercises, can increase mitochondrial content and capacity. Research using a standard strength training protocol revealed a regeneration of muscle mitochondria from a genetic perspective (Melov et al. 2007). Older individuals (average age of 68 years) who performed 24 weeks of basic resistance exercise had favorable mitochondrial adaptations in more than 175 genes associated with age and exercise. In fact, after 6 months of strength training, the older adults' mitochondrial characteristics changed so much that they were essentially the same as those of younger adults (average age of 24 years). These positive results led the researchers to conclude that resistance exercise can reverse specific aging factors in muscle tissue.

REVERSING PHYSICAL FRAILTY

Even people well past the age of 50 can benefit from sensible strength training. Several studies have shown that reasonable amounts of resistance exercise can enable elderly adults to regain strength, fitness, and physical abilities. In a study of nursing home residents (average age 88 years), we found significant improvements in measures of functional capacity and performance of daily living activities. The residents in this study performed 1 set of 6 resistance machine exercises with a weight load that permitted 8 to 12 controlled repetitions, 2 days a week (Mondays and Fridays) for a period of 14 weeks. These basic and brief exercise sessions produced remarkable results. On average, the previously frail study participants added 4 pounds of muscle and lost 3 pounds of fat, for a 7-pound improvement in body composition (Westcott 2009). They increased their leg strength by 80 percent and upper-body strength by 40 percent, enabling them to do less wheelchair sitting and more walking as well as other physical activities such as bicycling. Similar studies with frail elderly individuals have revealed additional resistance training benefits, such as greater movement control and faster walking speed.

COMBATING CANCER

Research from the University of Maryland indicates that resistance exercise may reduce the risk of colon cancer, which is the second leading cause of cancer deaths, by increasing the speed of food transport through our gastrointestinal system. However, the majority of studies on strength training and cancer have addressed the role of resistance exercise in cancer survivors. A comprehensive review of this research has shown that strength training is well tolerated by adult cancer patients and may provide a variety of health and fitness benefits during and after treatment. Most prominent among these benefits are reduced fatigue, increased muscle strength, improved body composition, and enhanced physical function (especially shoulder mobility in patients recovering from breast cancer). Although more research is needed in this area, it would appear that resistance exercise may play a preventive role in some types of cancer and may produce positive physiological responses during treatment and recovery periods in other types of cancer.

PRACTICAL APPLICATION

If we were to compare the muscles of the body to an automobile, they would be analogous to the engine. As noted earlier, your muscles serve as the engines of your body, and strong muscles enable you to function better in all physical activities. Your muscles are also similar to the shock absorbers and springs in an automobile, and strong muscles help you to feel better because they protect joints from a variety of potentially harmful external forces. Finally, muscles are like the chassis of an automobile because they largely define your appearance. Although excess fat can definitely detract from your appearance, your muscles actually provide your fundamental physique or figure. Consequently, strong muscles make you look better.

If you would like to function better, feel better, and look better, then you should begin a regular resistance training program that progressively strengthens all your major muscle groups. As you will learn in the following chapters, you can attain excellent results from relatively basic and brief programs of strength training using resistance machines in fitness centers or by performing free-weight or body-weight exercises in your home. We present research-based training protocols that are safe, effective, and efficient, with a proven track record of success for people over age 50.

Without regular resistance exercise you will continue to lose muscle and bone, and you will have further reductions in strength and fitness. Aerobic activity such as walking, running, cycling, and dancing are preferable for promoting heart health and cardiorespiratory fitness, but they will not prevent age-related reductions in muscle and bone. Continue to perform regular aerobic activity, but be sure to complement your endurance exercise with sensible strength training.

Likewise, sensible nutrition is essential for general health, and dieting is far and away the fastest way to lose body weight. However, excellent eating habits alone will not prevent the loss of muscle and bone or the continued weakening of your musculoskeletal system. Dieting can be particularly problematic because low-calorie diets decrease both fat weight and lean (muscle) weight. The undesirable muscle loss results in reduction of metabolic rate that makes it most difficult to maintain the lower body weight. In fact, research reveals that 95 percent of dieters regain all of the weight they lost within the year after their diet program (Mann et al. 2007).

However, as you may recall, the older adults in our nutrition and strength training study concurrently lost 9 pounds of fat weight and added 3 pounds of lean (muscle) weight, for a 12-pound improvement in their body composition over a 10-week period (Westcott et al. 2013). Be sure to eat healthy and nutritious foods, with a reasonable reduction in caloric intake if necessary, but do not diet without performing appropriate resistance exercise. Remember that muscle gain is positively associated with increased metabolism and decreased fat.

Ideally, you should adopt a lifestyle that includes sound nutrition (presented in chapter 12), regular aerobic activity, and sensible strength training. All of these complementary activities are essential for optimal health and fitness and especially for enjoying older adult years.

SUMMARY

Most athletes engage in resistance exercise to improve sport performance. These include older athletes who run, cycle, row, swim, ski, golf, play tennis, and engage in other physically challenging activities. However, most people over age 50 are at least as concerned about their general health and fitness as they are about their athletic abilities. This chapter presents 13 medically oriented and research-based reasons for engaging in regular resistance exercise:

1. Rebuilding muscle
2. Recharging metabolism
3. Reducing fat
4. Reducing resting blood pressure
5. Improving blood lipid profiles
6. Enhancing postcoronary performance
7. Resisting diabetes
8. Increasing bone density
9. Decreasing physical discomfort
10. Enhancing mental health
11. Revitalizing muscle cells
12. Reversing physical frailty
13. Combating cancer

Men and women of all ages respond favorably to sensible strength training, which has been shown to improve many health and fitness factors associated with quality of life and quantity of years. When you implement one of the strength training programs presented in this book, you take a proactive role in your personal health care. There is no medicine that provides as many physical and mental benefits as regular resistance exercise does.

Adapted from Westcott WL. Resistance training is medicine: effects of strength training on health. *Current Sports Medicine Reports* 11(4): 209-216, 2012, courtesy of the American College of Sports Medicine.

2

Assessment for Success in Training

You are ready to begin a program of strength training to develop more muscular ability and physical capacity. The logical place to start is to determine your muscular fitness level. However, before you do that, you should learn about factors that influence your muscular potential. After addressing these, we explain the process for determining your overall strength level, help you to select a program that is appropriate, and end the chapter with a discussion on the secrets of successful training. We recommend that before doing the strength assessments in this chapter you acquire your physician's approval for performing resistance exercise. Certain conditions may preclude your participation in a strength training program. In addition, the Assessing Your Physical Readiness questionnaire will help you determine whether you are physically ready to start strength training. You should complete this questionnaire before you begin training.

FACTORS THAT INFLUENCE STRENGTH POTENTIAL

The three most critical characteristics that affect your muscular fitness are sex, age, and lifestyle. Nonetheless, regardless of your sex, age, or lifestyle, the training programs in this book enable you to gain strength and add muscle to attain higher levels of physical fitness and functional ability. Let's take a closer look at these factors as they relate to strength development.

Sex

It is no secret that men are stronger than women. For example, in our study of more than 900 middle-aged adults, the men were found to be 50 percent stronger than the women in a standard test of leg strength. Does this mean that males have higher-quality muscle than females? Not at all. It simply means that men, who are typically larger, have more muscle mass than women. When compared on a muscle-for-muscle basis, however, the men and women in this study were equally strong. Research also reveals that men and women have similar rates of improvement in muscular strength and endurance even though women typically use lighter training loads (Castro et al. 1995). So the only real difference between men's and women's approaches to strength training is the amount of weight used.

ASSESSING YOUR PHYSICAL READINESS

If you answer yes to any of the following questions, you should talk with your doctor *before* beginning a weight training program.

YES   NO

_____ _____ Are you over age 50 (female) or 40 (male) and not accustomed to exercise?

_____ _____ Do you have a history of heart disease?

_____ _____ Has a doctor ever said your blood pressure was too high?

_____ _____ Are you taking any prescription medications, such as those for heart problems or high blood pressure?

_____ _____ Have you ever had chest pain, spells of severe dizziness, or fainting?

_____ _____ Do you have a history of respiratory problems, such as asthma?

_____ _____ Have you had surgery or problems with your bones, muscles, tendons, or ligaments (especially in your back, shoulders, or knees) that might be aggravated by an exercise program?

_____ _____ Is there a good physical or health reason not already mentioned here that you should not follow a weight training program?

From W. Westcott and T. Baechle, 2015, *Strength training past 50*, 3rd ed. (Champaign, IL: Human Kinetics). Adapted, by permission, from T.R. Baechle and R.W. Earle, 2014, *Fitness weight training*, 3rd ed. (Champaign, IL: Human Kinetics), 17.

Age

It has been well established that aging results in decreased muscle strength. In fact, among adults who do not perform resistance exercise, there is a decrease of 5 to 10 percent in strength every decade. This is caused by the gradual loss of muscle tissue that accompanies the aging process. Unless you strength train regularly, you lose several pounds of muscle every decade of adult life—typically 5 pounds (2.3 kg) for women and 7 pounds (3.1 kg) for men—which results in a lower strength level and a slower resting metabolic rate.

Lifestyle

Fortunately, regular resistance training maintains and increases muscle strength and muscle mass. Our research data provide reasonable estimates of average strength levels for men and women of various ages (Westcott 1994a; see table 2.1).

Table 2.1   Average Exercise Loads on Common Machines (*n* = 245)*

		AGE GROUPS					
Exercises		20-29	30-39	40-49	50-59	60-69	70-79
Leg extension							
Males	lb	112.5	105.0	97.5	90.0	82.5	75.0
	kg	51.0	47.6	44.2	40.8	37.4	34.0
Females	lb	67.5	65.0	62.5	60.0	57.5	55.0
	kg	30.6	29.5	28.3	27.2	26.1	24.9
Leg curl							
Males	lb	112.5	105.0	97.5	90.0	82.5	75.0
	kg	51.0	47.6	44.2	40.8	37.4	34.0
Females	lb	67.5	65.0	62.5	60.0	57.5	55.0
	kg	30.6	29.5	28.3	27.2	26.1	24.9
Leg press							
Males	lb	240.0	220.0	200.0	180.0	160.0	140.0
	kg	108.9	99.8	90.7	81.6	72.6	63.5
Females	lb	165.0	150.0	135.0	120.0	110.0	100.0
	kg	74.8	68.0	61.2	54.4	49.9	45.4
Chest cross							
Males	lb	100.0	95.0	90.0	85.0	80.0	70.0
	kg	45.4	43.1	40.8	38.6	36.3	31.8
Females	lb	57.5	55.0	52.5	50.0	47.5	45.0
	kg	26.1	24.9	23.8	22.7	21.6	20.4
Chest press							
Males	lb	110.0	102.5	95.0	87.5	80.0	72.5
	kg	49.9	46.5	43.1	39.7	36.3	32.9
Females	lb	57.5	55.0	52.5	50.0	47.5	45.0
	kg	26.1	24.9	23.8	22.7	21.6	20.4
Compound row							
Males	lb	140.0	132.5	125.0	117.5	110.0	102.5
	kg	63.5	60.1	56.7	53.3	49.9	46.5
Females	lb	85.0	82.5	80.0	77.5	75.0	70.0
	kg	38.6	37.4	36.3	35.2	34.0	31.8
Shoulder press							
Males	lb	105.0	97.5	90.0	82.5	72.5	62.5
	kg	47.6	44.2	40.8	37.4	32.9	28.3
Females	lb	50.0	47.5	45.0	42.5	40.0	37.5
	kg	22.7	21.6	20.4	19.3	18.1	17.0
Biceps curl							
Males	lb	90.0	85.0	80.0	75.0	70.0	60.0
	kg	40.8	38.6	36.3	34.0	31.8	27.2
Females	lb	50.0	47.5	45.0	42.5	40.0	37.5
	kg	22.7	21.6	20.4	19.3	18.1	17.0

(continued)

Table 2.1 *(continued)*

		AGE GROUPS					
Exercises		**20-29**	**30-39**	**40-49**	**50-59**	**60-69**	**70-79**
Triceps extension							
Males	lb	90.0	85.0	80.0	75.0	70.0	60.0
	kg	40.8	38.6	36.3	34.0	31.8	27.2
Females	lb	50.0	47.5	45.0	42.5	40.0	37.5
	kg	22.7	21.6	20.4	19.3	18.1	17.0
Low back							
Males	lb	110.0	105.0	100.0	95.0	90.0	85.0
	kg	49.9	47.6	45.4	43.1	40.8	38.6
Females	lb	80.0	77.5	75.0	72.5	67.5	65.0
	kg	36.3	35.2	34.0	32.9	30.6	29.5
Abdominal curl							
Males	lb	110.0	105.0	100.0	95.0	90.0	80.0
	kg	49.9	47.6	45.4	43.1	40.8	36.3
Females	lb	65.0	62.5	60.0	57.5	55.0	52.5
	kg	29.5	28.3	27.2	26.1	24.9	23.8
Neck flexion							
Males	lb	70.0	67.5	65.0	62.5	60.0	55.0
	kg	31.8	30.6	29.5	28.3	27.2	24.9
Females	lb	45.0	42.5	40.0	37.5	35.0	32.5
	kg	20.4	19.3	18.1	17.0	15.9	14.7
Neck extension							
Males	lb	80.0	77.5	75.0	72.5	70.0	60.0
	kg	36.3	35.2	34.0	32.9	31.8	27.2
Females	lb	52.5	50.0	47.5	45.0	42.5	40.0
	kg	23.8	22.7	21.6	20.4	19.3	18.1

Note that the loads shown in these charts have been established using Nautilus resistance machines and that using other equipment might result in slightly different results.

Reprinted, by permission, from T.R. Baechle and W.L. Westcott, 2010, *Fitness professional's guide to strength training for older adults*, 2nd ed. (Champaign, IL: Human Kinetics), 216-217. Adapted from W. Westcott, 1994, "Strength training for life: Loads: Go figure," *Nautilus Magazine* 3(4): 5-7, by permission of W.L. Westcott.

The estimates do not account for differing lifestyle choices, such as physical activity patterns. For example, if you have a physically demanding occupation, such as carpentry, you are likely to be stronger than a neighbor who is an accountant. Likewise, if you enjoy active hobbies, like gardening or hiking, you will probably be stronger than a friend who spends time knitting.

Although your lifestyle and activity patterns may influence your current strength level, they will not limit your potential for developing strength if you decide to start strength training. Whatever your beginning level of strength is, you can become a lot stronger than you are now. And that is what really matters—personal physical improvement that enhances your health, fitness, appearance, daily function, and sport or activity performance.

ASSESSING OVERALL MUSCULAR STRENGTH

We recommend three simple assessment procedures for evaluating your current level of muscular fitness. Based on the results of these assessments, you will choose the strength training program that is most appropriate for maximizing your rate of muscular development and minimizing the risk of unproductive or counter-productive exercise sessions.

Assessment of Upper-Body Strength

The first assessment procedure should be somewhat familiar because it involves the traditional push-up exercise. Push-ups, when properly performed, work the muscles of the chest (pectoralis major), back of the arms (triceps), and shoulders (deltoids) and serve as a relatively reliable predictor of upper-body strength. Perform the push-up test in the following manner.

Starting Position for Push-Up Test

- Men: Assume a standard push-up position with toes on floor, knees straight, body straight from heels to shoulders, head up, hands on floor slightly wider than shoulder-width apart, and elbows extended (see figure 2.1*a*).

- Women: Assume a modified push-up position with knees on floor, body straight from shoulders to hips, head up, hands on floor slightly wider than shoulder-width apart, and elbows extended (see figure 2.1*b*).

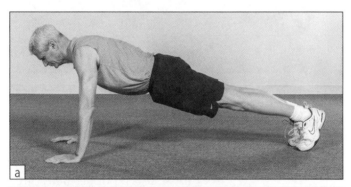

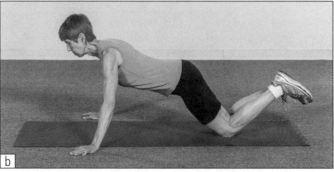

Figure 2.1   Push-up starting position: *(a)* standard for men and *(b)* modified for women.

Execution of Push-Up Test

- Lower your body slowly until your elbows form right angles and upper arms are parallel to the floor (see figures 2.2*a* and 2.2*b*). Keep your body straight, taking one full second for the downward movement.
- Push your body upward slowly until your elbows are fully extended. Keep your body straight, taking one full second for the upward movement.
- Inhale during the downward movement; exhale during the upward movement.

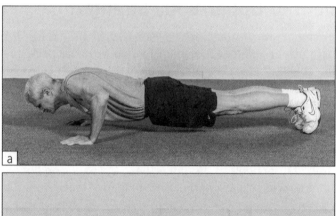

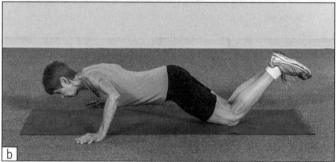

Figure 2.2 Push-up execution position: *(a)* standard for men and *(b)* modified for women.

Three Steps to Determining Upper-Body Strength

1. Perform as many push-ups as possible without straining yourself.
2. Record the number of consecutive push-ups completed with correct technique at the top of table 2.2.
3. Identify the number range your score falls into in the left column, and circle the corresponding number 5, 6, or 7 in the right column.

Table 2.2 Push-Up Classification Chart for Assessing Upper-Body Strength

NUMBER OF PUSH-UPS COMPLETED __		Upper-body strength index score (circle a number)
Men	Women	
0-9	0-9	5
10-19	10-19	6
20 or more	20 or more	7

A printable table 2.2 is available online at www.humankinetics.com/products/all-products/Strength-Training-Past-50-3rd-edition.

Assessment of Midsection Strength

Our second strength assessment also uses a familiar exercise, one that you may perform regularly. The trunk curl is a simple exercise that involves the abdominal muscles (rectus abdominis). When performed correctly, the trunk curl test provides an excellent evaluation of midsection, or core, strength and endurance. Perform the trunk curl test in the following manner.

Starting Position for Trunk Curl Test

- Lie faceup on the floor with your head, upper back, arms, and hips on the floor, hands next to hips, knees bent approximately 90 degrees, and feet flat on the floor (see figure 2.3*a*).

Execution of Trunk Curl Test

- Contract your abdominal muscles to lift your upper back and head off the floor as far as possible, typically 4 to 6 inches (10 to 15 cm) between shoulders and floor. Your lower back should remain in contact with the floor as your hands slide forward (see figure 2.3*b*). Take one full second for the upward movement.
- Lower your upper back and head to the floor, resuming the starting position. Take one full second for the downward movement.
- Do not drop quickly to the floor or bounce up from it.
- Exhale during the upward movement; inhale during the downward movement.

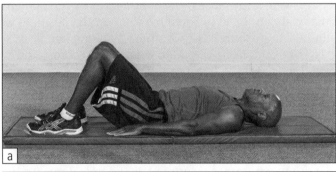

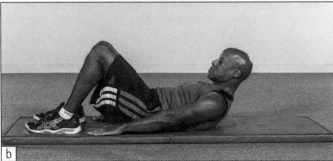

Figure 2.3   Trunk curl: *(a)* starting opposition and *(b)* execution.

Three Steps to Determining Midsection Strength

1. Perform as many trunk curls as possible.
2. At the top of table 2.3, record the number of consecutive trunk curls completed with correct technique.
3. Identify the number range your score falls into in the column on the left, and circle the corresponding number 5, 6, or 7 in the right column.

Table 2.3 Trunk Curl Classification Chart for Assessing Midsection Strength

NUMBER OF TRUNK CURLS COMPLETED __		Midsection strength index score (circle a number)
Men	Women	
0-24	0-19	5
25-49	20-39	6
50 or more	40 or more	7

A printable table 2.3 is available online at www.humankinetics.com/products/all-products/Strength-Training-Past-50-3rd-edition.

Assessment of Leg Strength

Unlike the push-up and trunk curl tests, which involve moving body weight, the leg strength test uses equipment. The YMCA leg extension test (Westcott 1987), which calls on the muscles in the front of the thigh (quadriceps), assesses lower-body strength. The exercise is easy to learn and perform safely.

To complete the YMCA leg extension test you need access to a leg extension machine. These are available in virtually all fitness clubs and are also common in home gyms.

A unique characteristic of the YMCA leg extension test is that it evaluates muscular strength relative to body weight; a person who weighs more is expected to be able to lift more weight. Because the score is based on the percentage of your body weight that you can lift 10 times rather than on the absolute weight of the load you lift, this test more fairly assesses strength among people of substantially varying weights. For example, a 100-pound woman who completes 10 repetitions with 50 pounds earns the same score as a 150-pound woman who completes 10 repetitions with 75 pounds because both women perform the exercise with 50 percent of their body weight.

The classification categories established for this test are based on the test results of more than 900 men and women with training experience. This test should give you a good indication of your lower-body strength and help you select your entry-level strength training program. Be sure to follow instructions for the YMCA leg extension test precisely as they are presented.

Starting Position for YMCA Leg Extension Test

Sit on the leg extension machine with your knee joints in line with the machine's axis of rotation (the point around which the movement arm revolves), back in full contact with the seat back, hands on the handgrips, and shins against the movement pad (see figure 2.4a).

Execution of YMCA Leg Extension Test

- Lift the movement pad upward until your knees are fully extended (see figure 2.4b). Take two full seconds for the upward movement.
- Pause momentarily with the knees fully extended in the up position.
- Lower the movement pad downward until the weight plate almost, but not quite, touches the remaining weight stack. Allow four full seconds for the downward movement.
- Exhale as you lift the movement pad upward, and inhale as you lower it.

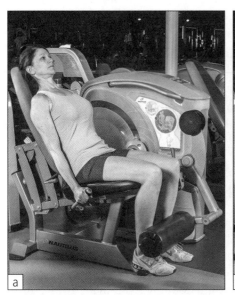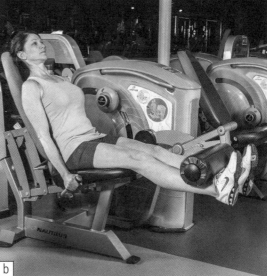

Figure 2.4   Leg extension: *(a)* starting position and *(b)* execution.

Six Steps to Determining Lower-Body Strength

1. Determine a load that is 25 percent of your body weight, insert the weight stack pin closest to that weight, and perform 10 repetitions. Rest 2 minutes.

2. Increase the load so that it is about 35 percent of your body weight and perform 10 repetitions followed by 2 minutes of rest.

3. Increase the load so that it is about 45 percent of your body weight and perform 10 repetitions followed by 2 minutes of rest.

Table 2.4 Leg Extension Classification Chart for Assessing Lower-Body Strength

SCORE FOR LOWER-BODY STRENGTH ___		Lower-body strength index score (circle a number)
Men	Women	
0-49%	0-39%	5
50-69%	40-59%	6
70% or higher	60% or higher	7

A printable table 2.4 is available online at www.humankinetics.com/products/all-products/Strength-Training-Past-50-3rd-edition.

4. Continue testing in this manner, progressively adding more weight, until you find the heaviest load that you can lift 10 times with correct technique.

5. Divide this load by your body weight to determine your lower-body strength score, and record this number in the blank provided in table 2.4. For example, if you weigh 120 pounds and you completed 10 leg extensions with 40 pounds, then your leg strength score is 33 (40 divided by 120 equals .33, or 33 percent).

6. Identify which range your score falls into in the column on the left, and circle the corresponding number 5, 6, or 7 in the right column.

DETERMINING OVERALL STRENGTH AND YOUR STRENGTH TRAINING PROGRAM

You can now use the strength index numbers circled in the far-right columns of tables 2.2, 2.3, and 2.4 to establish your overall strength. This information will tell you which of the strength training programs presented in chapters 9, 10, and 11 is best suited to your strength level and reason for training.

Simply add up the three numbers in the far-right columns and divide by 3. For example, if you scored 5 on all three tests, then your overall strength score is 5 (15 divided by 3 equals 5). If you scored 5, 5, and 6, then your overall strength score is 5.3 (16 divided by 3 equals 5.3). If you scored 7, 7, and 6, then your overall strength score is 6.6 (20 divided by 3 equals 6.6).

If your average score for the three strength tests is 5, 5.3, or 5.6, then you should begin with one of the strength training programs presented in chapter 9, Base Training Programs. If your average score for the three strength tests is 6, 6.3, 6.6, or 7, then you should begin with one of the strength training programs in chapter 10 (Advanced Training Programs) or the sport-specific programs in chapter 11. If your reason for strength training is to improve your performance in a sport and you are new to strength training and your score is 5, 5.3 or 5.6, be sure to start with one of the programs in chapter 9. We recommend that you follow one of the programs in chapter 9 for at least two weeks before selecting one of the sport-specific programs in chapter 11.

Although you may start training at a lower level than indicated by your overall strength score, we advise against beginning at a level higher than indicated by your overall strength assessment.

It is possible that you may not be able to perform one of the strength tests because of injury or inaccessibility to a leg extension machine. If you complete only two tests, add both strength index scores and divide by 2 to determine your overall strength score.

Like you, we take strength training seriously, and we want you to find an exercise program that is best suited to your current level of muscular fitness. By performing the three assessments in this chapter, you will acquire knowledge about strength in your upper body, midsection, and lower body that will help you determine which strength training program in chapters 9, 10, or 11 is best for you. It is worth the time and effort to evaluate your overall muscular strength because this information will help you to implement the most effective exercise program for further development of strength.

SECRETS OF EFFECTIVE TRAINING

Having determined your overall strength and which programs are most appropriate for your strength level, it is the ideal time to learn about the secrets of effective training. Although these suggestions may seem to be common sense, they can have a dramatic positive effect on your training experience. Read these guidelines and then go to chapter 9, 10, or 11 to begin training.

Train Regularly

You are virtually guaranteed success if you follow the workouts presented in this book—which means that you will be training on a regular basis. Sporadic training does not produce results! One of the most effective strategies is to work out with a partner. Being accountable to someone will make you train consistently; just find a partner who has a similar personal schedule and make plans to meet at a certain time on specific days.

Increase Workout Intensity Gradually

To allow your muscles time to adjust to the stress of weight training, adhere to the recommended number of training weeks described in each workout in chapters 9 to 11. Following the directions will allow you to gradually increase in intensity or difficulty of the workouts and allow for sufficient recovery to produce maximal results.

Eat Smart and Get Enough Rest

Do not underestimate the importance of nutrition and rest. Remember this training formula:

Regular training + balanced meals + adequate rest = dramatic improvements

Unfortunately, many people give attention to only one or two of these factors. If one is missing, the results of your program will be less than optimal. Although much has been written on the value of nutritional supplements, respected nutritionists continue to stress the importance of eating balanced meals (approximately 15 percent protein, 55 percent carbohydrate, and 30 percent fat). Research (Westcott and Loud 2013; Westcott et al. 2013) advocates the benefits of increased protein intake for people over age 50, especially when it is consumed before and after strength workouts, which is discussed along with sample meal plans in chapter 12.

While water has no calories and technically is not a food, it is by far the most important nutrient. The human body is mostly water (muscles are 80 percent water) and can survive only a few days without adequate hydration. The standard recommendation is to consume eight 8-ounce glasses of water daily; people who exercise need considerably more. Unfortunately, your natural thirst mechanism declines with age, so you should monitor your water consumption to ensure that you are well hydrated. Therefore, in addition to the eight 8-ounce glasses of water that you should drink each day, drink one or two more 8-ounce glasses of water on the days you weight train.

Also, because coffee, tea, diet drinks, and alcoholic beverages act as diuretics (which have a dehydrating effect), you should not count on these to provide your daily needs. But you may substitute beverages such as seltzer and fruit juices for water. Apple juice is an excellent source of potassium, and orange juice is high in vitamin C. Cranberry juice is close to orange juice in vitamin C content and may help prevent bladder infections. Carrot juice is high in vitamin A, vitamin C, potassium, and fiber.

Besides nutrition, your body needs rest in order to rebuild muscles after training as much as it needs training to stimulate improvement. Initially, you need to train two or three times a week. More is not always better. If you train too often, your muscles do not have enough time to recover, assimilate protein, and rebuild, and you might even injure yourself. Training smart means that you train regularly, eat balanced meals, get enough rest, and stay hydrated.

WARM-UP AND COOL-DOWN

Strength training is high-effort exercise that places relatively heavy demands on your musculoskeletal system. Therefore, you should not jump right into a strength workout, nor should you abruptly end a strength workout. Warm-up activities such as brisk walking or jogging in place for about 3 to 5 minutes will help you physically and mentally in training. You may also elect to include a few body-weight exercises such as knee bends, side bends, or trunk curls. For a warm-up procedure that will recruit the same muscles used in an exercise, perform 10 repetitions with half of the training load in each exercise as suggested at the beginning of chapters 9 to 11. After your workout, gradually decrease your activity level to let your body cool down and recover. This period is essentially a warm-up in reverse. It helps the muscular and cardiovascular systems gradually shift from a working to a resting state. The cool-down is particularly important for older adults because blood that accumulates in the lower legs after vigorous exercise can cause undesirable changes in blood pressure that may lead to cardiovascular complications. Five to 10 minutes of cool-down activities, such as easy walking and cycling followed by stretching exercises, will facilitate a smooth return to resting circulation and blood flow to the heart. Examples of four easy stretches are shown in figure 2.5. Hold each stretching exercise for approximately 15 seconds. While there may be a tendency to not commit time to the cool-down segment in workouts, it is an important transitional activity that should be a standard part of each training session.

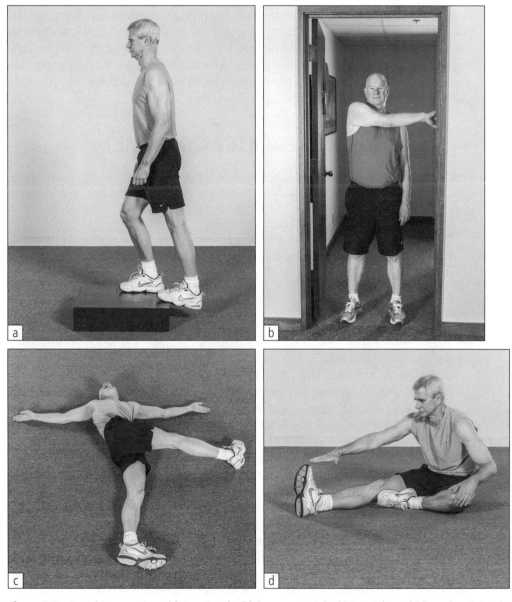

Figure 2.5 Stretching exercises: *(a)* step stretch, *(b)* doorway stretch, *(c)* T stretch, and *(d)* number 4 stretch.

WEIGHT TRAINING ATTIRE

Strength training is a challenging physical activity that requires functional exercise clothing. We recommend wearing loose-fitting shorts and a T-shirt or a lightweight warm-up suit. Loose and light exercise clothes enable you to easily transfer body heat to the environment, helping you avoid undesirable rises in body temperature. Proper activity wear also allows freedom of movement, permitting you to move comfortably and without restriction through a full range of exercise actions. Beyond your clothes, you should consider other attire such as shoes and gloves.

Wear athletic shoes that provide good traction and prevent slipping. Look for shoes that have a normal heel width (e.g., tennis shoes) rather than a waffle heel (running shoes). Cross-training shoes are ideal for strength training. Weight training gloves are not a necessity, but if you have trouble sustaining a firm grip, we recommend using them. When purchasing gloves, select those that have a leather palm and mesh back, are flexible, and fit snugly.

FITNESS FACILITY OR HOME?

You may decide that you need the environment of a fitness facility to enjoy the workouts presented in this book. If so, these are the key factors to consider when choosing a training center:

- Availability of exercise equipment
- Qualifications of the fitness staff
- Services offered
- Membership costs

Ideally, the facility you choose will be well equipped and will employ qualified professional instructors who can develop and implement a training program that meets your needs and fits your abilities. In addition, an exercise area should be spacious. Accidents are rare among adult strength trainers, but crowded exercise areas can increase the likelihood that accidents will occur. If you wish to train at a fitness center, choose one that has plenty of space between the strength training machines and free-weight equipment. Avoid facilities that have cluttered floors because items underfoot increase the potential for injury. In addition, too many people in the exercise room can hinder your concentration, possibly leading to mishaps.

For many people, training at home is the only practical option because of time constraints, membership costs at fitness facilities, or both. If you decide to train at home, find a spacious area to set up your exercise equipment and specific places to store the weights. Setting up workout equipment in a corner of a cluttered room can make your training sessions less enjoyable and create safety problems, especially if the exercise area is too small. Make sure you have ample lighting and air ventilation and at least one electrical outlet. An electrical outlet offers the opportunity to use a DVD or MP3 player, radio, TV, treadmill, or stepping machine. If practical, select a location with a high ceiling and that has carpet-covered concrete. Avoid training on tile or uncovered concrete floors because both can be slippery. Place equipment such as a bench and treadmill at least 18 inches (46 cm) apart to allow for easy access.

SELECTING A PERSONAL TRAINER

A knowledgeable personal trainer can help you enjoy and benefit the most from the training programs presented in this book. A good personal trainer is capable of individualizing the workouts presented in chapters 9 to 11, showing you how to perform the exercises correctly, and motivating you to make each workout most productive. If necessary, the trainer can also give you advice about the equipment you need for home use and recommend a reputable store where you can purchase the appropriate equipment at a reasonable price. If you decide to hire a personal trainer to help you with training, we strongly recommend that you identify one who has the skills just discussed and that you also ask prospective trainers the following questions. Then have the trainer provide you with references from current and previous clients.

- *Describe your academic preparation for personal training.* Look for course work associated with exercise physiology, biomechanics, nutrition, and, ideally, a degree in exercise science, exercise physiology, physical therapy, athletic training, or physical education.

- *What certification credentials directly associated with personal training have you earned?* Look for personal trainers who have earned certifications offered by organizations that are accredited by the National Commission for Certifying Agencies (www.credentialingexcellence.org/ncca), such as the National Strength and Conditioning Association (NSCA), American College of Sports Medicine (ACSM), and American Council on Exercise (ACE).

- *How long have you been a personal trainer?* Look for someone who has been active in the business of personal training for at least two years. Be cautious about hiring an inexperienced personal trainer.

Before signing a contract with a personal trainer, observe a prospective trainer working with a client. Even if you like what you see, delay signing a contract until you train with him or her for at least one session. Also, consider the cost, which typically ranges from $50 to $100 a session, and ask if the cost per session is less if you commit to a specific number of sessions.

MAINTAIN A POSITIVE ATTITUDE

It seems that nothing worthwhile comes easily, and this applies to weight training. However, if you make the commitment to train on a regular basis, the dramatic improvements in your appearance, fitness, and physical performance will convince you that it was a worthwhile investment of your time and effort. Every minute of every day invested in training makes a difference, so don't miss a training session unless you have a serious illness or injury. One missed session leads to two, two to three, and then what you could have achieved will not happen. Develop the attitude that the hour you put aside for training is the time that you are doing something for yourself. It is your time, so be protective of it and productive with it. You will feel better about yourself physically and mentally. Weight training is the one thing that you can do in an hour that will positively affect appearance, fitness status, health, and performance. Your investment in training time will yield rich rewards.

SUMMARY

This chapter has helped you determine your muscular fitness level and identify which programs in chapters 9 to 11 are most appropriate for you. You've also discovered the secrets of successful training. If you are new to strength training and desire to undertake a sport-specific training program in chapter 11, it is important that you follow one of the beginning programs in chapter 9. Following the recommendations provided in this chapter will make your training enjoyable, safe, and productive. Chapter 3 focuses on principles that will make your training safer and bring about positive changes in your muscular fitness in an efficient manner.

3

Applying Principles of Training

In this chapter, we present research-based guidelines that are essential for maximizing strength development and ensuring a safe training experience. These guidelines are discussed in the following order: variables of program design, exercise technique, and organization of workouts.

The need to address program design should be obvious, and this section examines all essential training factors. However, it is equally important to address proper exercise technique and the need for warm-up and cool-down periods because they are related to your training effectiveness and decreasing the risk of injury. Finally, you should find the information on organization of the workout helpful, especially if you intend to undertake strength training and aerobic training during the same workout.

VARIABLES OF PROGRAM DESIGN

This chapter provides guidelines for selecting and organizing exercises and for determining training frequency, weight loads to use, number of repetitions and sets to perform, and the length of rest periods between sets and exercises. The chapter also explains how to maximize your training effort and outcome. Adhering to these guidelines will result in a safe and successful strength training experience.

Exercise Selection

Hundreds of strength training exercises can be performed with free weights (barbells, dumbbells, kettlebells), weight-stack machines, exercise balls, resistance bands, and body-weight resistance. It is therefore important to carefully select exercises that provide the best balance of exercise effectiveness, training efficiency, and workout safety. This section presents the rationale for designing a purposeful and practical program of strength exercises that will bring about comprehensive muscle development in accordance with sensible principles of training.

Perform One Exercise for Each Major Muscle Group One of the most important guidelines for choosing exercises to include in your program is to perform at least one exercise for each major muscle group (i.e., chest, shoulders, back, arms, core, and legs). Doing so ensures that your workouts will result in symmetrical muscular development. As you can see in the left column of table 3.1, there is at least one exercise for each major muscle group.

Select Exercises for Opposing Muscle Groups   Many people select certain exercises because they are more popular, more convenient, or more satisfying to perform than others. For example, most strength training programs feature bench presses for upper-body development. It is true that the bench press strengthens the muscles of the chest, front of the shoulder, and back of the arm (triceps). However, if you do not give equal attention to the opposing muscles of the upper back, back of shoulder, and front of the arm (biceps), you may develop a strength imbalance that leads to poor posture and a greater susceptibility to joint injuries.

opposing muscles—Muscles that produce opposing movements around a joint (e.g., biceps that bend the elbow and triceps that straighten it).

strength imbalance—Disproportionate strength on one side of a joint or muscle area as a result of overemphasizing the training on one side.

Order of Exercises

There seems to be general confusion about the order in which strength exercises should be performed. Some people prefer to begin workouts with their stronger muscle groups, and others choose to start training their weaker muscle groups while they are fresh. Because larger muscle groups (e.g., quadriceps, or anterior thigh) use more energy, produce more fatigue by-products, and elicit higher blood pressure responses than smaller muscle groups (e.g., biceps), most strength training authorities recommend an exercise order that progresses from larger to smaller muscle groups.

We prefer to train larger muscle groups before smaller muscle groups. Table 3.1 lists the major muscle groups from largest (thigh) to smallest (forearms) and suggests an order for performing exercises that develop each of these muscle groups: lower-body exercises, followed by upper-body exercises, followed by those for the core (midsection) and neck. Some refer to this as priority training because it prioritizes exercises that work the larger muscles before the smaller muscles. Arranging the order of exercises in this manner ensures that you train the larger muscles while you are fresh, enabling you to emphasize their development over smaller groups.

Of course, you do not have to use this recommended sequence for training. For example, you may occasionally want to work your weaker muscle groups first while you are fresh. Keep in mind, though, that when you vary the order of exercises, the number of repetitions you can perform will change accordingly. You should be able to perform more repetitions of an exercise if you move it from the end to the beginning of your training session, because you will be less fatigued in the early stages of your workout.

Training Frequency

Regular strength training stresses your muscles and produces some degree of tissue microtrauma. After each workout, the exercised tissues respond to the training stimulus by rebuilding tissue, resulting in larger and stronger muscles. These tissue-building processes typically take 48 to 96 hours. Although your training frequency may vary, most people make consistent strength improvements with two or three exercise sessions per week.

Table 3.1   Suggested Exercises for Major Muscle Groups

Muscle group	Machine exercise	Free-weight exercise	Alternative exercise
Front thigh (quadriceps)	Leg extension	Dumbbell squat or barbell squat	Wall squat with exercise ball
Rear thigh (hamstrings)	Leg curl	Dumbbell squat or barbell squat	Back squat with resistance band
Inner thigh (hip adductors)	Hip adduction	—	—
Outer thigh (hip abductors)	Hip abduction	—	—
Lower leg (gastrocnemius)	Heel raise	Dumbbell heel raise	—
Chest (pectoralis major)	Chest crossover	Dumbbell or barbell bench press	Chest press with resistance band
Upper back (latissimus dorsi)	Pullover	Dumbbell one-arm row	Seated row with resistance band
Shoulders (deltoids)	Lateral raise	Dumbbell seated press	Seated shoulder press with resistance band
Front arm (biceps)	Biceps curl	Dumbbell standing curl	Biceps curl with resistance band
Rear arm (triceps)	Triceps extension	Dumbbell overhead triceps extension	Bench dip with exercise ball
Low back (erector spinae)	Low back extension	Body-weight trunk extension	—
Abdominals (rectus abdominis)	Abdominal flexion	Body-weight trunk curl	Trunk curl with exercise ball
Sides (external and internal obliques)	Rotary torso	Twisting trunk curl	Twisting trunk curl with body weight
Front neck (sternocleidomastoids)	Neck flexion	—	—
Rear neck (upper trapezius)	Neck extension	Dumbbell or barbell shrug	Shrug with resistance band
Forearms (wrist flexors and extensors)	Forearm flexion and extension	Wrist curl and extension	

An every-other-day strength training program (e.g., Monday–Wednesday–Friday or Tuesday–Thursday–Saturday) ensures consistency and produces excellent results. But two strength workouts a week produce nearly as much muscle development as three strength workouts a week. As shown in figure 3.1, in our 8-week study of 1,132 participants, those who trained two days a week had almost 90 percent as much muscle development as those who trained three days a week (Westcott and Guy 1996). Our follow-up 10-week study, also shown in figure 3.1, involving 1,644 participants revealed equal gains in muscle weight for those who trained two days

tissue microtrauma—Temporary weakening of muscle cells that stimulates tissue-building processes and strength development.

a week and those who trained three days a week. The average age of the trainees in both of these studies was over 50, so these findings are applicable to our recommended training protocols (Westcott et al. 2009).

Based on these studies, we recommend two or three strength training sessions a week. Your rate of muscle development should be about the same whether you do two or three weekly workouts. Although you can gain strength by training only one day a week, your rate of muscle development will be reduced by about 50 percent, based on our research (Westcott et al. 2009).

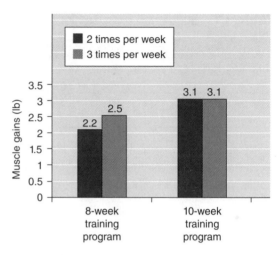

Figure 3.1 Changes in lean (muscle) weight for men and women performing two or three strength training sessions a week (2,776 participants).

Another fact to remember is that consistency is as important as frequency. Missing scheduled training sessions is unproductive, and training your muscles two days in a row to make up for a missed session is counterproductive. Therefore, you should establish a regular strength training workout schedule that is compatible with your lifestyle and includes either two or three nonconsecutive days of training each week.

Exercise Sets

An exercise set refers to a group of consecutive repetitions that you perform in a given exercise. For example, if you pick up the dumbbells and perform 10 biceps curls, then return the dumbbells to the rack, you have completed one set of 10 repetitions. If you rest and then repeat this procedure, you have completed two sets of 10 repetitions. People starting a strength training program should perform one set of each exercise.

One set of an exercise is the minimum required for strength improvement, and single-set strength training is an efficient means of muscle development. One research study (Westcott, Greenberger, and Milius 1989) on upper-body strength gains—measured by increases in repetitions performed—showed similar results among groups of participants who did one, two, or three sets of chin-ups and bar dips over a 10-week training period (see figure 3.2).

A University of Florida study (Starkey et al. 1996) compared

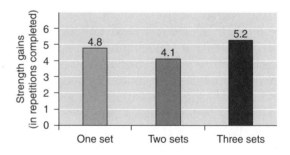

Figure 3.2 Comparison of one-, two-, and three-set strength training (77 participants).

lower-body strength gains—measured by percentage of increase in the load lifted—for participants who performed one or three sets of leg extensions and leg curls. As illustrated in figure 3.3, both training groups made almost equal gains in lower-body strength during the 14-week training period. Based on the results of these studies, it seems both prudent and productive to begin strength training with one set of each exercise and then progress to two or three exercise sets if you have the time and motivation to do so.

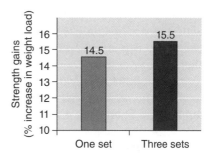

Figure 3.3 Comparison of one- and three-set strength training (38 participants).

Rest Periods Between Sets and Exercises

When performing two or more sets of the same exercise, allow your muscles to recover for one to two minutes between sets. This is sufficient time to rest your muscles and restore most of your anaerobic energy supply. Also take a brief rest between successive exercises to reduce the general effects of fatigue on subsequent muscular efforts. Resting about one minute between different exercises as you progress through your workout is usually sufficient.

Exercise Load

The first safety concern for anyone participating in strength training is to select an appropriate exercise resistance, or load. The most important consideration is ensuring your beginning weight loads are not too heavy. Of course, the weight, load, or amount of resistance you use largely determines the number of repetitions that you can perform in an exercise set.

For example, if your strength assessment in chapter 2 places you in the chapter 9 training programs, then you will use loads that enable you to complete 12 to 16 repetitions of the exercises listed.

If you begin with one of the workouts in chapter 10, you will use heavier loads that enable you to complete 8 to 12 repetitions in some of the exercises and 4 to 8 in the more advanced workouts. Generally speaking, most people can complete 16 repetitions with approximately 60 percent of their maximal load, 12 repetitions with approximately 70 percent of their maximal load, 8 repetitions with approximately 80 percent of their maximal load, and 4 repetitions with approximately 90 percent of their maximal load. For example, if your exercise range is 8 to 12 repetitions, start with a load that enables you to comfortably perform 8 to 10 repetitions. Continue training with this load until you can complete 12 repetitions using proper technique, then increase the resistance in accordance with the overload principle.

For decades, successful strength training programs have been built on the overload principle. Overload means using progressively heavier loads to stimulate further strength development. For example, if you can complete 10 bench presses with 100 pounds, you could experience an overload by simply increasing the weight by 5 pounds and performing as many repetitions as you can with this slightly heavier load.

It is possible to apply the overload principle by performing low repetitions with relatively heavy loads or by performing a high number of repetitions with relatively light loads. Therefore, guidelines are necessary. These guidelines are based on the percentage of the maximum amount of weight that you can lift in an exercise one time, referred to as percentage of maximum resistance. Because of the stable relationship between resistance and repetitions presented in the following section, it is not necessary for you to determine your maximum weight loads. Charts are also provided in each of the program chapters (9, 10, and 11) to help you select the appropriate exercise resistance. For most training purposes, you should use loads that allow you to perform 4 to 16 repetitions, which equals 90 to 60 percent, respectively, of the maximum load you can lift one time.

Relationships Between Maximum Resistance and Repetitions

Maximum resistance, generally referred to as the repetition maximum or 1RM weight load, is the heaviest resistance that you can lift one time. Loads that are less than 100 percent of 1RM will permit the number of repetitions shown in the following list.

95 percent 1RM = 2 repetitions

90 percent 1RM = 4 repetitions

85 percent 1RM = 6 repetitions

80 percent 1RM = 8 repetitions

75 percent 1RM = 10 repetitions

70 percent 1RM = 12 repetitions

65 percent 1RM = 14 repetitions

60 percent 1RM = 16 repetitions

In a study examining relationships between resistance and repetitions (Westcott 2002), 141 participants were tested to determine how many repetitions they could complete with 75 percent of their maximum resistance. As illustrated in figure 3.4, the average number of repetitions performed was 10.5. However, some people performed fewer repetitions and some performed more repetitions using the same relative load. These differences are caused by genetic variations in muscle fiber makeup, and they explain in part why some people prefer lower-repetition training and others prefer higher-repetition training.

Exercise Repetitions and Loads

The key to developing stronger muscles is using a progressive training system that gradually increases the loads used in each exercise. Loads that allow you to perform

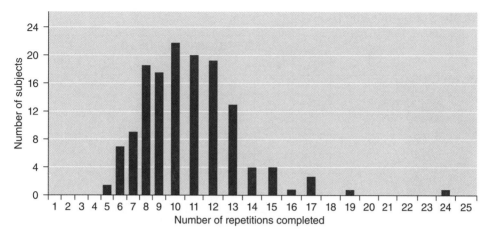

Figure 3.4 Distribution of repetitions completed with 75 percent of maximum weight load (141 participants).

4 to 16 reps using your best effort are considered ideal. If you select a load that is too heavy, you will not be able to complete 4 reps. If it is too light, you will be able to perform more than 16 reps. As muscles become stronger in response to training, using the same load will result in more repetitions. When this occurs, it is important to increase the load, which creates the overload that is needed to stimulate further increases in strength. Table 3.2 provides steps for identifying how much to increase training loads if the amount of weight used is too heavy or too light.

1. In chapter 9, 10, or 11, determine how many repetitions you should perform.
2. Go to table 3.2 (left column) and locate and circle the repetition range.
3. Under the heading "Repetitions completed," highlight the repetition range that includes the number of repetitions that you were able to complete with the load used.
4. Where the "Repetition range" row and "Repetitions completed" column intersect is the load adjustment you should make.
5. Correct the training load for your next workout by decreasing (–) or increasing (+) the original load accordingly.
6. Repeat this procedure as needed; sometimes you might have to make several adjustments to get the right training load.

For example, the number of repetitions listed for the workout selected is 10 in the bench press exercise, and you performed 15 repetitions with 110 pounds. The load is too light. In the left column of table 3.2, 10 repetitions fall within the repetition range of 10 to 11. To identify the load change needed, find where this horizontal line intersects with the 14 to 15 "Repetitions completed" column. Where these lines intersect, a +10 is shown. When you add 10 to the original 110-pound load, the adjusted load is 120 pounds.

Generally speaking, it is advisable to periodically progress from higher-repetition training with lighter loads to lower-repetition training with heavier loads and then

Table 3.2 Adjusting Loads

		REPETITIONS COMPLETED									
		>18	16-17	14-15	12-13	10-11	8-9	6-7	4-5	2-3	<2
Repetition range	14-15	+10	+5		−5	−10	−15	−15	−20	−25	−30
	12-13	+15	+10	+5		−5	−10	−15	−15	−20	−25
	10-11	+15	+15	+10	+5		−5	−10	−15	−15	−20
	8-9	+20	+15	+15	+10	+5		−5	−10	−15	−15
	6-7	+25	+20	+15	+15	+10	+5		−5	−10	−15
	4-5	+30	+25	+20	+15	+15	+10	+5		−5	−10
	2-3	+35	+30	+25	+20	+15	+15	+10	+5		−5

Reprinted, by permission, from T.R. Baechle and R.W. Earle, 2014, *Fitness weight training*, 3rd ed. (Champaign, IL: Human Kinetics), 34.

repeat the process as your training becomes more advanced. As an example, the sample base training programs in chapter 9 use 12 to 16 repetitions, while the more advanced programs in chapter 10 uses heavier loads resulting in 8 to 12 repetitions or as few as 4 to 8 repetitions. After several weeks using 4- to 8-repetition training, consider reducing the weight loads and switch to higher-repetition sets (12 to 16 reps or 8 to 12 reps) for a couple of months before progressing again to fewer repetitions with heavier loads.

Loads for Resistance Band Exercises   Unlike barbells, dumbbells, or the weight stack of a machine, the difficulty or intensity level of a resistance band does not rely on gravity. Instead, it depends on the thickness of the band and how far it is stretched. Many (but not all) band manufacturers follow a color progression of yellow (thinnest and easiest to stretch), red, green, blue, black, silver, and gold (thickest and hardest to stretch). Be aware, though, that there are other color bands such as pink, maroon, light blue, orange, and brown that may have varying ranges of thickness. Because there is not a standard weight or load for resistance bands, it is difficult to determine which one (color) to start with or progress to when you are ready to increase the difficulty of an exercise. The best approach to selecting the correct load when using resistance bands is to identify the recommended number of repetitions in the workouts in chapters 9, 10, and 11 and then, through trial and error, find the band that results in that number of repetitions.

Loads for Kettlebell Exercises   Because many kettlebell exercises involve multiple muscle groups, it can be difficult to determine training loads. The weight selected depends on your level of fitness and the exercise. Again, the best approach to selecting the correct load when using kettlebells is to identify the recommended number of repetitions in the workouts in chapters 9, 10, and 11 and, through trial and error, find the kettlebell that results in that number of repetitions.

Training Progression

As you continue training, you will increase your muscular strength and want to use heavier weight loads. Progression is the key to continued strength development, but you must approach it gradually and systematically for best results. Keep in mind that strength training is a lifetime activity, and there is no reason to do too much too soon, which can lead to injury and setback.

Double-Progressive System   We recommend the 5 percent rule, which you can easily apply to any of the strength training protocols in this book, for safe and successful progression of strength training. The 5 percent rule dictates that whenever you can complete the number of reps in the upper end of your repetition range during two successive workouts, you should increase the resistance by 5 percent (or less) in your next workout. For example, if you are using a protocol of 12 to 16 repetitions, and you complete 16 leg extensions with 100 pounds in two successive workouts, you should raise the resistance to 105 pounds for your next training session. Likewise, if you are using a protocol of 8 to 12 repetitions, and you complete 12 reps with 50 pounds twice in a row, you should raise the resistance by 2.5 pounds in your next workout.

This is a double-progressive system in which you first increase the number of repetitions (within the desired rep range) performed and then add resistance (by 5 percent or less). Although relatively simple in application, this double-progressive approach has an outstanding safety record and typically enables beginning participants to attain more than 40 percent gains in strength after just two months of training.

Multiple-Set Training   Another strategy for progressively increasing the workout intensity is the use of multiple-set training. Multiple-set training offers a greater volume of muscular work for each exercise and may be performed by people who prefer a longer training session. Within this approach are three standard protocols.

1. Use the same training load in all sets and perform the same number of repetitions.
2. Increase the training load in each set and perform the same number of repetitions.
3. Increase the load in each set and reduce the number of repetitions.

In the first approach, you perform multiple exercise sets with the same training load, such as completing three sets of 10 leg extensions using 100 pounds for each set. This exercise protocol provides both a relatively high training volume and a relatively high training effort on each exercise set, making it a challenging workout when using appropriate resistance.

In the second example, you follow an exercise protocol that features multiple-set training with increasingly greater loads, such as a set of 10 leg extensions with 60 pounds, a second set of 10 leg extensions with 80 pounds, and a third set of 10 leg extensions with 100 pounds. This training method provides a progressive warm-up before performing the heaviest set, but it requires a relatively high training effort on only the final exercise set.

In the third option, you follow a training method, sometimes referred to as the pyramid approach, which involves using heavier loads and fewer repetitions in successive sets. For example, you perform 10 leg extensions with 100 pounds, 8 leg extensions with 115 pounds, and 6 repetitions with 130 pounds. A well-designed pyramid protocol requires a relatively high training effort in each exercise set and involves the use of relatively heavier weight loads than the other training methods. If you are a less experienced exerciser, you should probably begin multiple-set training with protocol 2 because it provides progressive warm-up sets and only one high-effort set. If you are more experienced, you may choose either protocol 1 or protocol 3, depending on whether you prefer to perform high-effort sets with the same resistance or high-effort sets with progressively heavier weight loads and correspondingly fewer repetitions.

Because a wide range of exercise loads can produce excellent strength gains, periodically train with different percentages of your maximum load. For example, the sample programs in chapter 9 use 60 to 70 percent of maximum resistance (12 to 16 reps), and those in chapter 10 use 70 to 80 percent (8 to 12 reps) and 80 to 90 (4 to 8 reps) percent of maximum resistance. Systematically changing your exercise resistance offers both physiological and psychological benefits. Keep in mind that strength training with loads of 60 to 90 percent of maximum is highly effective for gaining strength and building muscle.

Training Effort

Exercise physiologists agree that training at a high level of muscular effort enhances strength development. You'll get the best results when your exercise intensity is high enough to fatigue the target muscles. This level of fatigue will occur if you train to muscle failure in each set. Following this guideline and performing 4 to 16 repetitions with 90 to 60 percent, respectively, of your maximum load will provide an ideal training effect. As your strength improves, you should also consider ways to increase your exercise effort.

For example, you may perform a set of leg extensions, rest one or two minutes, and complete another set of leg extensions. As a more efficient alternative, you may perform a set of leg extensions followed closely by a set of leg presses. Both of these exercises target your quadriceps muscles but involve different movement patterns to provide an additional training stimulus. Of course, you should follow this more challenging type of workout only if you want to put greater effort into your exercise program.

ORGANIZATION OF WORKOUT

Now that you understand how to choose and sequence exercises and how to determine weight loads and repetitions, let's examine how to best organize your workout. This section presents information about performing aerobic (cardiorespiratory) exercise in the same workout as strength training. It also provides guidelines for warming up and cooling down.

Strength training is best for improving muscular fitness, and aerobic exercise is best for improving cardiorespiratory fitness. But if you want to include both activities in the same training session, is it better to begin with strength training or endurance exercise?

In one of our studies (Westcott and Loud 1999), 205 adults performed identical programs of strength training (10 machines) and endurance exercise (25 minutes of cycling, walking, or stepping) three days a week for 10 weeks. Half of the participants always did the strength training first, and half of the participants always did the endurance exercise first. As presented in table 3.3, both training groups had essentially equal increases in strength after two months of exercise. Therefore, the order in which you perform strength training and aerobic exercise is largely a matter of personal preference. Of course, if your primary goal is to improve muscular fitness, it makes sense to perform strength training first. If your main objective is better cardiorespiratory fitness, it is logical to perform endurance exercise first.

Table 3.3 Strength Gain and Workout Order

Training protocol (10 weeks)	Mean weight increase for 10 Nautilus machines (in pounds/kilograms)
Strength exercise first	+16/7.3
Endurance exercise first	+15/6.8

Whichever order of activities you choose, be sure to begin each training session with a few minutes of warm-up exercise (refer to chapter 2) and conclude each training session with a few minutes of cool-down exercise. These transition phases between rest and vigorous physical activity provide important physiological and psychological benefits.

SUMMARY

The components of the strength training program discussed in this chapter are selection, order, training frequency, sets, rest periods, loads, repetitions, training progression, and training effort. With a practical understanding and appreciation of these training principles, you are now prepared to design safe and productive strength training programs. Continued improvement requires the right training intensity, which is most affected by loads, reps, and the number of sets performed. Finally, consider the order in which exercises are organized, or ordered, in your workouts and the importance of warming up and cooling down. All of these considerations for strength training are presented in table 3.4 with recommendations for successful performance and program implementation. To derive the benefits of strength training while reducing the likelihood of injury, we recommend that you adhere to these guidelines.

Table 3.4 Summary of Principles and Practices of Strength Training

Variables of program design
Exercise selection: Select at least one exercise for each major muscle group to create symmetrical muscular development. Choose exercises that train opposing muscles groups to ensure a strength balance across joints and muscle areas.
Exercise order: Train your lower body first, then your upper body, followed by core and neck exercises; work the larger muscles in these body areas first.
Training frequency: Train on 2 or 3 nonconsecutive days each week.
Exercise sets: Begin your strength training program with 1 set of each exercise. As you become more advanced, consider adding a second or third set of exercise if you so desire.
Rest periods between sets and exercises: Rest 1 to 2 minutes between sets of the same exercise, and rest 60 to 90 seconds between different exercises.
Exercise load: For most training purposes, use a load that allows you to lift 4 to 16 repetitions. This corresponds to 90 to 60 percent of your maximum resistance, respectively.
Exercise repetitions: Depending on the training loads used, perform 4 to 16 repetitions in each set of exercises.
Training progression: Raise training loads about 5 percent whenever you complete the prescribed number of repetitions with proper form during two successive workouts. Progress from more repetitions with lighter loads to fewer repetitions with heavier loads, then repeat the process. You may increase your training effort by performing more sets of exercises or by increasing the number of exercises for a given muscle or muscle group.
Training effort: Train to the point of momentary muscle failure in each set to derive maximum benefits, and consider making the workouts more challenging by adding more sets.
Factors of exercise technique
Movement speed: Perform all strength training exercises at slow to moderate speeds and always under control. A good guideline is to use 4 to 6 seconds for each repetition (2 to 3 seconds lifting and 2 to 3 seconds lowering).
Range of motion: Whenever possible, perform exercises through a full range of motion of the joint, from a position of full muscle stretch to a position of complete muscle contraction.
Breathing pattern: Breathe continuously during each repetition, exhaling through the more difficult (lifting, pushing, pulling) movement phase and inhaling during the easier (lowering and return) movement phase.
Organization of workout
Order of strength and aerobic workouts: Perform strength training and aerobic exercise in the order you prefer.
Warm-ups and cool-downs: Precede strength training sessions with 5 to 10 minutes of warm-up activity to gradually shift from rest to vigorous exercise. Conclude workouts with 5 to 10 minutes of cool-down activity.

4

Strength Training Equipment

The strength training equipment used in the programs in this book includes only a few of the hundreds of equipment options that are available to you. And because there are so many types of exercise equipment, for use both in the home and in fitness facilities, this chapter provides information on selecting the best resistance equipment for safe, effective, and efficient strength training. This chapter presents considerations for evaluating free-weight, machine, and alternative (resistance bands and exercise balls) exercise equipment and provides checklists to help you assess the safety and function of equipment.

FREE WEIGHTS

Other than resistance bands, the least expensive and most versatile equipment to purchase are free weights, including dumbbells, barbells, and kettlebells. Free weights do not take up much space, and you can use them to perform hundreds of exercises. The unrestrained movement patterns permitted by free-weight equipment allow your joints to move through their full range, thus increasing your flexibility and improving your overall muscle coordination. These advantages help explain why the use of free weights is so popular.

Let's look at the basic free-weight equipment you'll need if you choose this equipment option. Typically it will include a set of dumbbells, a barbell, a bench with supports, and perhaps some kettlebells.

Dumbbells

Adjustable dumbbells enable you to assemble the loads you need by adding weight plates to the dumbbell bar and securing them with locks, which are fasteners that fit on the ends of the bar. Make sure that the locks are easy to tighten and loosen and that you can rely on them to keep the weight plates securely on the bar.

Before purchasing locks, determine how much strength it takes to tighten and loosen them. Then, check to see if the weight plates stay on the dumbbell bar when it is tilted to a 45-degree angle. Ask the salesperson to tilt a lightly loaded bar to see if the weight plates stay on the end of the bar. If you do not have the grip strength required for easily using a particular type of lock, or if the weight plates slide off when the bar is tilted, seek a different type.

If you are willing to spend a little more money, the premolded, or fixed-weight, solid dumbbells are easier to use than the adjustable dumbbells (see figure 4.1). Because you do not have to assemble or disassemble them between exercises, premolded dumbbells enhance training efficiency. The downside of this type of dumbbell is that you need to purchase quite a few of them if you want to use various weight loads in your workouts, which you probably will.

A more economical approach, and one that will equip you with what you need to complete all of the exercises in the program

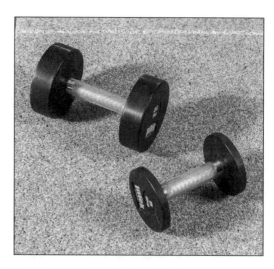

Figure 4.1 Premolded dumbbell.

options in chapters 9 to 11, is to purchase two adjustable dumbbells and the weight plates listed in the box titled Basic Dumbbell Set. Two dumbbells and 75 pounds (~35 kg) of weight plates provide 15 load options, ranging from 2 to 39.5 pounds (~1 to 18 kg) on each dumbbell, assuming an unloaded bar weighs 2 pounds (just under 2 kg), for approximately $80 (all costs are in U.S. dollars). Please note that the metric conversions listed are approximate conversions because there are no exact equivalents of metric weights to Imperial weights. For example, we list .5 kg as the metric version of the 1.25-pound weight plate, even though .5 is equal to only 1.1 pounds. There is no metric weight plate that corresponds to 1.25 pounds. The equipment listed will accommodate your needs for dumbbell equipment.

Basic Dumbbell Set

A basic adjustable dumbbell set includes the following (if you use the metric unit of measure, the nearest equivalents appear in parentheses):

- 2 dumbbell bars with locks and
- 4 of each of the following weight loads:
  - 10-pound (4.5 kg) plates
  - 5-pound (2 kg) plates
  - 2.5-pound (1 kg) plates
  - 1.25-pound (.5 kg) plates

Barbells

The barbell you select should be 5 or 6 feet (1.5 or 1.8 m) in length unless you prefer an Olympic barbell set that features a 7-foot (2 m) bar and revolving sleeves on which the weight plates are placed. As with dumbbells, easy-to-use but secure locks are essential. Therefore, apply the same convenience and safety criteria when selecting barbell locks. The list in the box titled Basic Barbell Set specifies the weight plates that compose a basic 100-pound (45 kg) barbell set. Most bars weigh 25 to 30 pounds (11.4 to 13.6 kg) when unloaded. Adding two 1.25-pound (.5 kg) plates to this set will provide more load options. The bar and plates specified create 16 load options at a cost of approximately $100.

Basic Barbell Set

A basic adjustable barbell set includes the following (if you use weights in metric units of measure, the nearest equivalents appear in parentheses):

- 1 barbell 5 to 6 feet (1.5 to 1.8 m) long with locks and
- 4 of each of the following weight loads:
    - 10-pound (4.5 kg) plates
    - 5-pound (2.5 kg) plates
    - 2.5-pound (1 kg) plates
    - 1.25-pound (.5 kg) plates

Kettlebells

A kettlebell resembles a cast-iron ball (like a cannonball) with a handle attached to the top of it (figure 4.2). It can weigh as little as 9 pounds (4 kg) or more than 100 pounds (45 kg). It is different from a dumbbell because the weight of the kettlebell is distributed unevenly, requiring your muscles to work harder to maintain your balance. You can perform standard weight training exercises with kettlebells such as the double bent-over row and front squat (see chapter 7). An advantage of kettlebell training

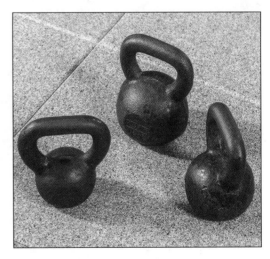

Figure 4.2 Standard kettlebells.

is that their use allows you to train multiple muscle groups at the same time, requiring muscle groups to work cooperatively, thereby improving overall muscle coordination. Training with kettlebells also results is an excellent whole-body workout.

Weight Benches

Weight benches are typically of two types: with and without uprights. Uprights provide a safe resting place for a barbell to be placed before and after a set of exercises. A flat bench does not have uprights (figure 4.3*a*), whereas a bench press (figure 4.3*b*) does. Both types of benches enable you to perform a variety of chest, arm, and shoulder exercises while lying on your back or while seated. If you intend to use one of the free-weight programs in chapter 9, 10, or 11, you'll need a bench-press bench to do the chest-pressing exercises with a barbell. A flat bench works fine for the basic free-weight workouts performed with dumbbells.

For a little more money you can purchase an incline bench that will adjust to various angles as shown in figure 4.3*c*. Because you can change the back pad to various positions, it is the most versatile type of bench for pressing exercises.

Certain exercises for the legs (e.g., squat) and shoulders (e.g., overhead press), and back of the arms (e.g., lying triceps extension) require one or more spotters so that you can perform the exercises safely. Using the type of squat rack shown in figure 4.4 will enable you to safely perform these without a spotter. So if you intend to include such exercises in your training programs and will not have someone spotting you, be sure to purchase a squat rack with safety bars.

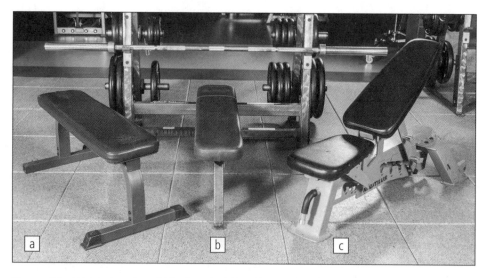

Figure 4.3   Weight benches: (*a*) flat bench; (*b*) bench press bench with uprights; (*c*) incline bench.

Costs for Free-Weight Equipment

The equipment requirements and costs associated with performing the free-weight exercises in chapters 9, 10, and 11 are presented in the box titled Costs for Basic and Optional Equipment later in this chapter. As indicated, the cost of the dumbbells and bench needed in the free-weight programs in this book is approximately $200, and the additional cost for equipment needed for the free-weight workouts is $680. Purchasing this equipment can provide several training options in your home for a relatively small initial investment. In comparison, a high-quality, easy-to-use, and versatile strength training machine costs $1,500 to $2,500.

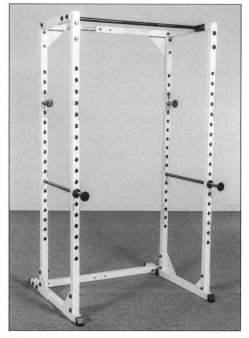

Figure 4.4 Squat rack.

Safety for Free-Weight Equipment

If you decide to purchase and exercise with free weights, use the Safety Checklist for Free Weights to safely achieve the most training benefit from your equipment. Time spent inspecting your equipment is always a good investment for ensuring safe and effective exercise sessions.

Safety Checklist for Free Weights

- Always load each end of the bar evenly.
- Make sure loose locks are secure and tight.
- Store weight plates appropriately so that you don't trip over them.
- Ensure that the bench is stable.
- Lift with your legs, not your back, when moving dumbbells and barbells from the floor to the racks.

Costs for Basic and Optional Equipment

Weight training equipment can range from inexpensive elastic bands to expensive machines. For your convenience, we list the approximate costs of the dumbbell and barbell equipment just discussed, and follow this discussion with information about kettlebells and elastic bands.

BASIC EQUIPMENT

For the free-weight exercises in chapters 9, 10, and 11 you'll need the following:

    2 adjustable dumbbells with locks and 75 pounds (~34 kg) of weight plates $80

    1 flat bench $130

    Total $210

    1 5-foot (1.5 m) barbell with locks; 25 pounds (11.4 kg) and 75 pounds (~34 kg) of weight plates $100

    1 bench-press bench (with uprights) $160

    1 squat rack $420

    Total $680

KETTLEBELL EQUIPMENT

If you choose to incorporate kettlebell exercises into your training program, you will need the following equipment:

    One of each of the following kettlebells: 15, 20, 25, 30, 35 pounds (kettlebells exist in metric increments of 6.5, 1.5, 8, 10, 12, 14, 16 kg)

    Total $125

OPTIONAL EQUIPMENT

    1 set of each of premolded (solid) dumbbell pairs (5, 10, 15, 20, 25 pounds, or the closest equivalents of 2.5, 4.5, 7, 10, 12 kg) $140

    1 adjustable bench (substitute for other benches) $160

    Total $300

Working With a Spotter

Some free-weight exercises, such as the barbell bench press, barbell squat, lying triceps extension, and barbell heel raise, increase your risk of injury because of the positioning of the barbell and the movement pattern. For example, if you are unable to complete the last repetition in the barbell bench press exercise and cannot place the barbell back on the standards, the bar might drop onto your chest or face and cause injury. Spotters can also help you lift the bar from the uprights to start an exercise, offer encouragement, and catch a barbell or dumbbell if you lose control of it or lose your balance, thus protecting you from injury. Having a spotter help you with free-weight exercises involving barbells or dumbbells held overhead (e.g., standing press), over the face (e.g., bench press, lying triceps extension), and on the back (e.g., squat, heel raise) is very important to your safety. These exercises and others requiring spotters are identified in chapter 7.

WEIGHT-STACK MACHINES

The popularity of strength training among men and women, which now exceeds 60 million in the United States, has spawned tremendous development of weight training machines, especially for use in home gyms (Kreuger 2004). Machine exercises have been designed for ease of performance and safety. You can change weight loads quickly, and movement patterns are predetermined, making machine exercises easier to perform than free-weight exercises. Machines also provide support for the body, and some models automatically match the resistance levels to your strength levels throughout the range of motion.

If you have problems with balance or are beginning at a low level of strength, start your strength training program using machines and the machine workouts described in chapter 9. Resistance machines allow you to do most of your exercises from a sitting position, usually with back support, or while lying faceup (see figure 4.5). They generally limit your movements to those actions that are unlikely to result in injury and to movement patterns that are appropriate for the target muscles. They eliminate the possibility of dropping barbells, dumbbells, kettlebells, or weight plates on yourself, and they don't require you to stoop to lift equipment. Once your balance is good and your strength levels are high enough, consider using free weights and following the free-weight workouts as well as the more advanced machine workouts in chapters 10 and 11 while following the standard safety precautions. Both types of equipment are well suited to bringing about dramatic improvements in your strength.

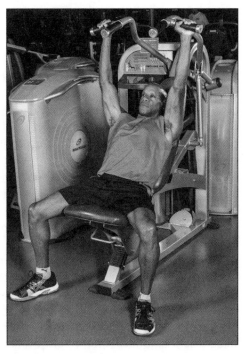

Figure 4.5 Machine equipment allows you to do most exercises while in a sitting position.

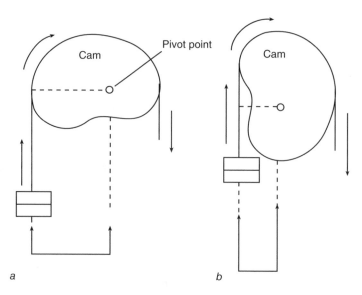

Figure 4.6 As the cam rotates from position 1 to 2, the distance from the pivot point to the weight plate shortens, which has the effect of reducing the load, resulting in a more uniform muscle effort throughout each repetition.

Reprinted, by permission, from T.R. Baechle and B. Groves, 1992, *Weight training: Steps to success* (Champaign, IL: Human Kinetics), 22.

Characteristics of Machines

Well-designed machines place a relatively consistent stress on the muscles by means of a cam or other device that creates a longer (figure 4.6a) or shorter (figure 4.6b) distance between the pivot point and point where the force is being applied, called the pivot-point distance. The design of the cam or other device is an attempt to match the shortest pivot-point distance with the most difficult range of the exercise and the longest pivot-point distance with the easiest range. Thus, the cam's shape attempts to match the strength curve (variation in strength throughout a range of motion) of the muscles involved in an exercise. In doing so, these machines provide a resistance that approximates a muscle's force capability at each angle of movement, enabling it to maintain a more consistent level of effort throughout each repetition.

Free-weight exercises involve leverage changes that produce more resistance in some exercise positions and less in other positions. For example, as the dumbbell in figure 4.6 reaches position 3, the distance between the elbow and the dumbbell and the force required to continue the curling movement are at their most challenging position. When fatigue terminates a repetition in this exercise, failure usually occurs at position 3 even though you have sufficient strength to continue curling the dumbbells from points 1 to 2 and 4 to 5. Well-designed machines attempt to accommodate your muscles' force capabilities, enabling them to contract through the most challenging position, referred to as the sticking point. When shopping for a machine, keep in mind that devices that use elastic resistance, such as those commonly advertised on television, may not effectively adapt to your muscles' varying capabilities. Their advantages over machines with cams and weight stacks, like those shown in figure 4.5, however, are that they are easy to move and store and are less expensive.

If you prefer to train on a machine in your home, consider the following points:

- Application—how easy the exercises will be to learn and execute
- Versatility—how many exercises you can perform on it
- Simplicity—how simple it is to set it up for different exercises
- Durability—quality of construction
- Convenience—ease of assembly and disassembly
- Reputation—status of the equipment manufacturer and of the distributor from which you intend to purchase the equipment
- Cost—price of the equipment, including shipping and installation

Machine Safety

If you decide to follow a machine training program, use the Safety Checklist for Machines to safely attain the most benefit from your equipment. If mechanical deficiencies exist, be sure to have them fixed before you use the equipment.

Develop training procedures that stress caution. Always fasten the seat belt if one is provided to ensure proper body alignment. And develop the habit of double-checking the little things. For example, if you use machines, learn the proper positioning of your seat and the correct load for each exercise; double-check them before each set.

Safety Checklist for Machines

- Check for frayed cables, belts, and pulleys; worn chains; and loose pads.
- Make sure plates move smoothly on guide rods.
- Adjust levers and seats as needed.
- Insert selector keys all the way into the weight stack.
- Keep your hands away from the chains, belts, pulleys, and cams.
- Never place your fingers or hands between weight stacks.

RESISTANCE BANDS

An alternative to machine and free-weight equipment is the use of resistance bands that are made of rubber tubing or elastic cable to create resistance as they are stretched (figure 4.7). Exercising with resistance bands is a convenient and practical choice if you cannot afford a fitness club membership or other strength training equipment, have limited space at home, or travel a lot. Resistance bands come in various lengths, types of handles, and colors; the latter indicates the relative degree of elasticity, or resistance. Many manufacturers of resistance bands use the same colors to indicate the amount of thickness (and thus the resistance to stretching) of their bands, starting with yellow as the thinnest and easiest to stretch and progressing in thickness to red, green, blue, black, silver, and gold. Some things to keep in mind when using resistance bands include the following:

1. Be aware of old, worn, or cracked bands that may break at the worst moment during a repetition.
2. Check that handles are securely attached to the rest of the band before performing an exercise.
3. When using a doorknob or piece of furniture to anchor one end of the band, be sure that no one will open the door and that the band is firmly affixed to the furniture and that the furniture will not move.

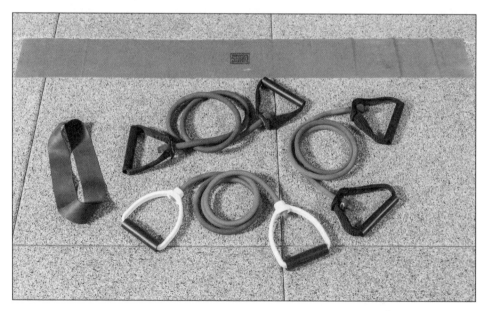

Figure 4.7 Various types of resistance bands.

EXERCISE BALLS

An exercise ball—sometimes referred as a stability ball, balance ball, body ball, fitness ball, physioball, or Swiss ball—is an air-filled ball made of soft vinyl and nylon with a diameter of about 22 to 30 inches (55 to 75 cm). Performing exercises on an exercise ball typically recruits more core muscle groups (lower back, abdominals, obliques) than when performing the same exercises on the floor, while standing, or while sitting on a bench. Although exercising on a less stable base usually requires using lighter resistance, involving the stabilizing muscle groups in addition to the target muscles adds a different dimension to standard exercises. Some things to keep in mind when performing exercises on an exercise ball include the following:

1. Be sure that the ball is fully inflated (especially with exercises that require the ball to support your body weight).

2. Select the correct size of ball for your height. When you sit on top of the ball with your feet flat on the floor, your thighs should be parallel to the floor. Refer to table 4.1 to assist you in determining the correct size of ball.

Table 4.1   Selection of Exercise Balls

Height of exerciser	Ball diameter
5 feet 1 inch to 5 feet 7 inches (155-170 cm)	55 cm (21.6 inches)
5 feet 8 inches to 6 feet 1 inch (173-185 cm)	65 cm (25.5 inches)
6 feet 2 inches to 6 feet 7 inches (188-201 cm)	75 cm (29.5 inches)

SUMMARY

Using the right equipment can add variety and enjoyment to your strength training as well as provide better results. Whether you decide to use machines, free weights, or other options, you should carefully consider the unique characteristics of each, and you should consult with qualified professionals before purchasing equipment. Regardless of the training equipment selected, heed the safety checklists provided in this chapter.

Learning Basic Exercise Techniques

Weight training is more than simply finding a barbell and pumping iron. This chapter outlines some dos and don'ts that will help you train safely and get the most out of the time and effort that you devote to training. You should read this chapter and understand the basics of proper weight training technique before you actually begin doing the exercises. In addition, knowing how to prepare to work out (the warm-up) and how to relax gradually after working out (the cool-down) will go a long way toward making each session successful (discussed in chapter 2).

LEARN LIFTING FUNDAMENTALS

Although weight training exercises number in the hundreds, several guidelines are universal: Use a good grip, establish a stable body position, and use effective techniques when picking up and putting down barbells, dumbbells, kettlebells, and even weight plates. You must also know how to breathe correctly during exercises.

Gripping a Barbell, Dumbbell, Kettlebell, or Handle

Grasping a dumbbell, kettlebell, or handle (machine and resistance band exercises) involves one consideration (pronated or supinated type of grip), whereas gripping a barbell involves two considerations (type of grip and grip spacing).

The two basic grips used with dumbbells, kettlebells, and handles are referred to as pronated (or overhand) or supinated (or underhand). When training with barbells, three grips can be used: pronated, supinated, and mixed (alternated) grip. As shown in figure 5.1a, in the overhand grip, palms face down, knuckles face up, and thumbs face toward each other. In the underhand grip (see figure 5.1b), palms face up, knuckles face down, and thumbs point away from each other. In the alternated grip (see figure 5.1c), one hand is in an underhand grip (palms facing up) and the other in an overhand grip (palms facing down) so your thumbs point in the same direction. To simplify your understanding of the proper grips to use in the exercise descriptions in chapters 6 to 8, reference is made to where the palms of your hands face (e.g., palms face up, palms face down, palms face each other, or palms face away).

All grips shown in figure 5.1 are closed grips, meaning that your fingers and thumbs are wrapped (closed) around the barbell or dumbbell bar, kettlebell grip, or handle. In an open grip, sometimes referred to as a false grip, your thumbs do not wrap around the bar. The open grip can be dangerous because the bar might

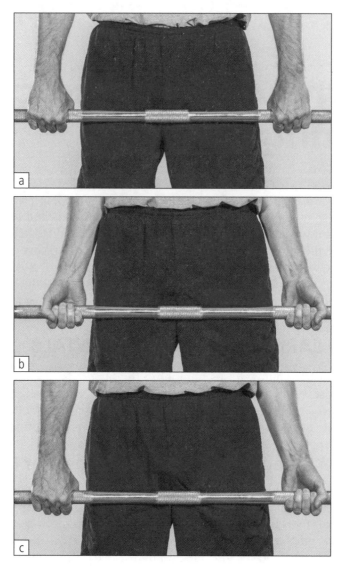

Figure 5.1 Types of grip: *(a)* pronated (overhand, in which palms face down); *(b)* supinated (underhand, in which palms face up); and *(c)* mixed (alternated, in which one palm faces up and the other faces down).

roll off your palms and onto your face or foot and cause severe injury. Always use a closed grip when weight training.

Several grip widths are used when training with barbells. In some exercises, your hands are placed about shoulder-width apart at an equal distance from the weight plates. Some exercises require a narrower grip than this, such as hip width. Other exercises require a wider grip. Figure 5.2 shows various grip widths. When reading the descriptions of the exercises in chapters 6, 7, and 8, be sure to note the type of grip and also the grip width in chapter 7 (free-weight exercises) for each exercise. Incorrectly placed hands can create an unbalanced grip and result in serious injury.

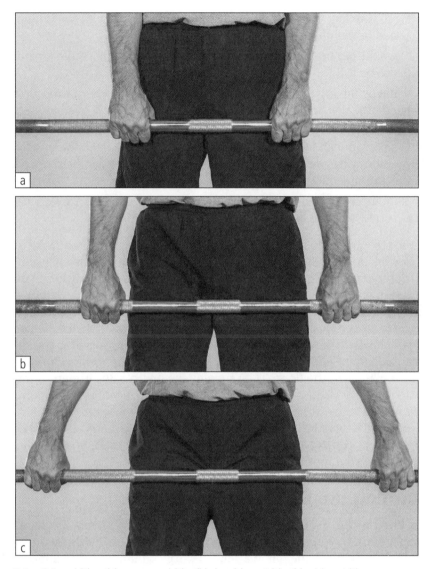

Figure 5.2   Grip widths: *(a)* narrow width; *(b)* shoulder width; *(c)* wide width.

Lifting the Bar off the Floor

Correctly lifting the bar (or any weight) off the floor is important to your safety. Improper lifting can place a significant amount of stress on your neck, upper and lower back, and knees; that stress can result in a serious injury. Establishing (getting into) a stable body position with a balanced and secure base of support is especially important for all standing exercises—especially overhead or squatting exercises with barbells, dumbbells, or kettlebells. While the following discussion involves a barbell, the guidelines provided apply to lifting any heavy object off the floor:

- Place your feet flat on the floor, shoulder-width apart, with your toes pointing ahead or slightly outward.
- Move the bar next to your shins (or as close as you can if there are no weight plates on it).
- Squat by flexing both your knees and your hips (in other words, do not just bend over at your waist) and grasp the bar with a closed, overhand, shoulder-width grip.
- Position your shoulders over the bar and establish a flat back (not rounded) position with your shoulders held back, chest out, head held up, and eyes looking straight ahead.
- Stand up with the bar and think, *Keep the bar close, use the legs, keep hips low, and keep the back flat, not rounded.*

The photo sequence in figure 5.3 shows how to lift a barbell safely. Take a look at the photos before reading the next section that describes the five phases.

The preparatory lifting position (figure 5.3a) places your body in a stable position, one in which your legs—not your back—will do the lifting. Getting into the proper position is not as easy as you might think. As you squat, one or both heels will tend to lift up, causing you to step forward to catch your balance. Remember to keep your heels on the floor! If a mirror is available, watch yourself as you squat into the low preparatory position. Does your back stay in a flat position? Do your heels stay in contact with the floor? They should (see figure 5.3b). The most important point to remember when you lift a barbell, dumbbell, weight plate, or any object off the floor is to use your leg muscles, not your back muscles.

If you need to pull the bar to your shoulders, continue pulling it past your knees (figure 5.3c), but do not allow the bar to rest on your thighs. As you straighten your legs and hips, your hips should move forward (figure 5.3d).

Returning the Bar to the Floor

When lowering the bar or any heavy object to the floor, remember to keep the bar or weight close to you and to keep your back flat and rigid, relying on your legs to squat down to move the bar in a slow, controlled manner to the floor. If the bar begins at shoulder height, allow the weight of the bar to pull your arms out and down, an action that will cause the bar to press against your thighs. Hold the bar briefly at midthigh before squatting to lower the bar farther to the floor. Remember to keep your head up and back flat throughout the return of the bar to the floor. In many ways, you will perform the movements described in figure 5.3 but in the reverse order.

Inexperienced exercisers tend to use momentum-assisted repetitions and an abbreviated range of motion to complete the desired number of repetitions. Accelerating the movement of the bar or handle during a repetition increases momentum and the likelihood of injury and reduces training effectiveness. Exercises that are not performed through the proper range of motion also decrease training effectiveness.

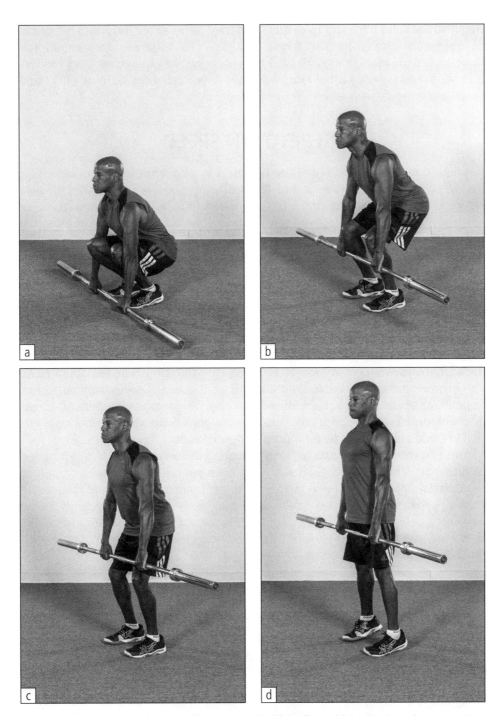

Figure 5.3 Proper technique for lifting a barbell off the floor: *(a)* getting into the preparatory lifting position; *(b)* using your legs to lift the bar (called the first pull); *(c)* pulling the bar past your knees and moving your hips forward (called the scoop or transition); *(d)* standing straight up with the bar at your mid-thigh, but not resting on it.

Beginners also tend to hold their breath as they perform the most difficult phase of the exercise movement, which results in higher blood pressure responses. The three technique guidelines presented next for repetition speed, range of motion, and breathing patterns are all important for maximizing the training effect and making your workouts safer.

REPETITION SPEED

Repetition speed refers to the time required to perform each repetition. This includes the total time you use to lift and lower the load (note that lift also refers to the upward direction that the weight stack, barbell, dumbbell, or kettlebell moves, regardless of the direction your body moves). Although the repetition speed during repetitions is partly a matter of personal preference, it is important to perform all exercise repetitions under control. *Under control* generally refers to repetitions that take at least 4 seconds to complete. These slow repetition speeds involve more muscular tension and less momentum, which should increase your training stimulus and decrease your risk of injury. But it is difficult to determine an ideal repetition speed for performing strength training exercises.

For example, a study examined the effects of 4-, 6-, 8-, and 14-second repetitions on strength development in 198 men and women (Westcott 1994b; see table 5.1). All four exercise groups made excellent strength gains over an 8-week training period. Repetition speeds of 4 to 14 seconds were all effective in improving strength across 13 major muscle groups. So there is clearly a range of controlled repetition speeds that are safe and productive for muscular development.

You can exert more muscular force lowering the weight load than lifting the weight load. Therefore, to challenge your muscles during the lowering part of the exercise, slow your repetition speed. For example, a popular and time-tested training protocol is 2 to 3 seconds for the lifting phase and 2 to 3 seconds for the lowering phase of each repetition. The training protocols in our program chapters use lifting and lowering speeds of 2 to 3 seconds each, thereby completing each repetition in about 4 to 6 seconds.

Table 5.1 Repetition Speed and Strength Improvement

Training protocol (8 weeks)	Reps per set	Time per set (in seconds)	Mean weight increase (on 13 Nautilus machines in pounds/kilograms)
4 sec/rep	10	40	+22/10
6 sec/rep	10	60	+22/10
8 sec/rep	10	80	+23/10.4
14 sec/rep	5	70	+27/12

One way to assess your repetition speed is the stop test. If you can stop the repetition at any point in the movement range during a repetition, you are using the right speed. Try this test during workouts to see if you are performing repetitions at the proper speed.

RANGE OF MOTION

We recommend exercising through the full range of joint motion for two reasons. First, research indicates that full-range strength training enhances joint flexibility. Second, studies show that full-range exercise movements are necessary for developing full-range muscular strength.

The importance of full-range muscular strength is underscored by extensive research on patients with low back pain (Jones et al. 1988). The researchers discovered that people with weak low back muscles were more likely to have low back pain than people with strong low back muscles. They also determined that exercising the low back muscles through their full range of motion was necessary for developing strength in all positions between full trunk flexion and complete trunk extension. This was an important finding because about 80 percent of the patients who increased their full-range back strength had less low back discomfort.

Although some people believe that strength training reduces joint flexibility, our research with golfers over age 50 showed that 8 weeks of full-range strength training exercises did not decrease their range of motion (Westcott, Dolan, and Cavicchi 1996). In fact, the golfers significantly improved their club-head speed and driving power as a result of the strength training program.

Full-range strength training exercise means training from the position of full muscular stretch to the position of full muscular contraction. Note that when the target muscle group (e.g., biceps) is fully contracted, the opposing muscle group (e.g., triceps) is fully stretched, and vice versa. Of course, you should not exceed normal joint limits or have pain in any portion of the exercise movement. Eliminate or abbreviate exercises that cause joint discomfort, training only in the pain-free range of motion.

BREATHING PATTERN

Regardless of the exercise, never hold your breath when strength training. Holding your breath may cause excessive internal pressure that restricts blood flow, resulting in lightheadedness and high blood pressure responses. Prevent these undesirable occurrences by breathing continuously during every exercise set. Exhale during the more difficult lifting, pushing, or pulling phase, sometimes referred to as the sticking point, and inhale during the easier lowering or return phase of each repetition.

Exhaling during the most difficult phase of a repetition and inhaling afterward will help maintain a more desirable internal pressure response. Because continuous breathing is a critical component of safe strength training exercise, practice proper breathing on every repetition.

SUMMARY

The grips described and illustrated in this chapter will enable you to correctly perform the exercises in chapters 6, 7, and 8. The techniques for lifting and lowering weight will help you avoid back injuries. The recommendations regarding speed of repetitions and range of motion are important for making the performance of the exercises in later chapters safe and will maximize your training results. Using the correct breathing pattern during the performance of all repetitions to avoid becoming dizzy or fainting is an essential technique in making training safe.

6

Machine Exercises

In chapters 1 to 4 you learned about the many benefits of strength training, how to assess your current strength training status, which training programs in this book are suited to you, keys to training success, and equipment that you will be using. In chapter 5 you learned about grips, stance and body positioning, speed of movement, and breathing techniques, all of which you will apply when performing the 26 machine exercises in this chapter.

As you review the machine exercises in this chapter and the free-weight and alternative exercises in chapters 7 and 8, you will note that some exercises are performed in a rotary movement pattern. That is, the exercise action is circular in nature. Rotary movements, such as leg extension and barbell curl, involve a single-joint action that is typically produced by one or sometimes two major muscle groups. For example, the leg extension exercise addresses the quadriceps muscles and activates the knee joints. Similarly, the barbell curl exercise addresses the biceps muscles and activates the elbow joints.

Other exercises are performed in a linear movement pattern. That is, the exercise action is essentially a straight line. Linear movements, such as leg press and bench press, involve more than one joint action and are typically produced by two or more major muscle groups. For example, the leg press exercise addresses the quadriceps, hamstrings, and gluteal muscles and activates both the knee and hip joints. Likewise, the bench press exercise addresses the pectoralis major, anterior deltoids, and triceps muscles and activates both the shoulder and elbow joints. We believe that a comprehensive strength training program should include both rotary and linear exercises to maximize overall muscle development.

LEG EXTENSION
Quadriceps

Beginning Position

1. Adjust seat so that knees are in line with machine's axis of rotation (where the machine pivots). The axis of rotation is indicated by a red dot on Nautilus machines, which are shown in the following exercise photos.
2. Sit with back firmly against seat back.
3. Position ankles behind roller pad, knees flexed about 90 degrees.
4. Grip handles.

Upward Movement Phase

1. Push roller pad slowly upward until knees are extended.
2. Exhale throughout upward movement.

Downward Movement Phase

1. Return roller pad slowly to starting position.
2. Inhale throughout lowering movement.

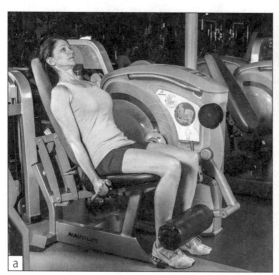
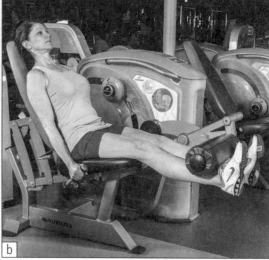

LEG CURL
Hamstrings

Beginning Position
1. Lie facedown on a bench with head in line with body.
2. Position ankles under roller pad with knees in line with machine's axis of rotation.
3. Grip handles.

Upward Movement Phase
1. Pull roller pad slowly upward until knees are fully flexed.
2. Exhale throughout pulling movement.

Downward Movement Phase
1. Allow roller pad to return slowly to starting position.
2. Inhale throughout return movement.

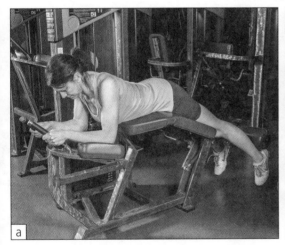 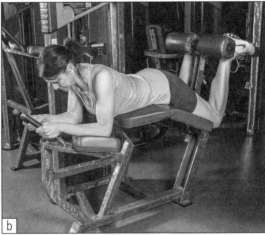

LEG PRESS
Quadriceps, hamstrings, gluteals

Beginning Position

1. Adjust seat so that knees are flexed to 90 degrees or less.
2. Sit with back firmly against seat back.
3. Place feet flat on foot pad in line with knees.
4. Grip handles.

Forward Movement Phase

1. Push foot pad forward slowly until knees are almost extended but not locked.
2. Keep feet, knees, and hips aligned.
3. Exhale throughout pushing phase.

Backward Movement Phase

1. Allow foot pad to slowly return to starting position.
2. Inhale throughout return movement.

Leg Exercise

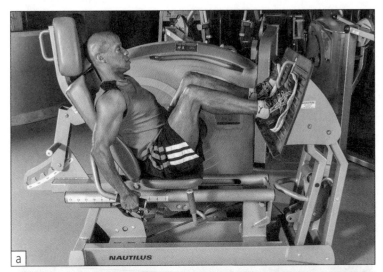

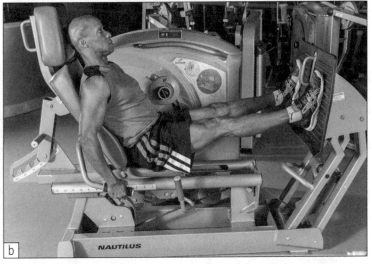

HIP ADDUCTION
Hip adductors

Beginning Position

1. Sit with back firmly against seat pad.
2. Position knees outside of movement pads and feet on supports.
3. Adjust movement lever to starting position with legs comfortably apart.
4. Grip handles.

Inward Movement Phase

1. Pull movement pads together slowly.
2. Exhale throughout pulling movement.

Outward Movement Phase

1. Allow pads to slowly return to starting position with legs apart.
2. Inhale throughout return movement.

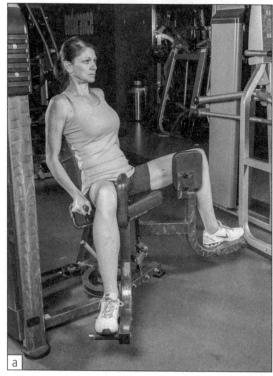
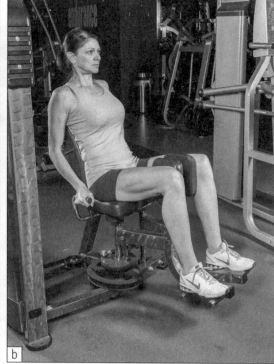

HIP ABDUCTION
Hip abductors

Beginning Position

1. Sit with back firmly against seat pad.
2. Position both knees inside of movement pads and feet on supports with legs together.
3. Grip handles.

Outward Movement Phase

1. Push movement pads apart slowly as far as comfortable.
2. Exhale throughout pushing movement.

Inward Movement Phase

1. Allow movement pads to slowly return to starting position with legs together.
2. Inhale throughout return movement.

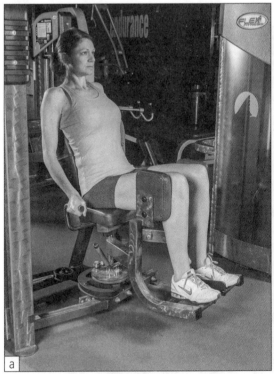
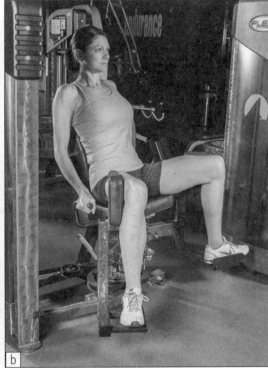

HEEL RAISE
Gastrocnemius, soleus

Beginning Position

1. Position and secure the resistance belt around waist.
2. Stand with balls of feet on rear edge of step.
3. Place hands on support bar.
4. Allow heels to drop below step as far as comfortable.

Upward Movement Phase

1. Rise slowly on toes to lift heels upward as high as possible.
2. Keep knees straight.
3. Exhale throughout upward movement.

Downward Movement Phase

1. Return slowly to starting position, heels below step.
2. Inhale throughout downward movement.

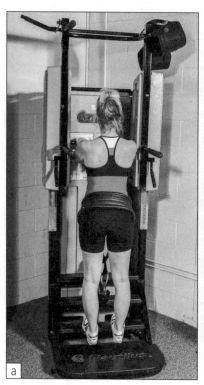 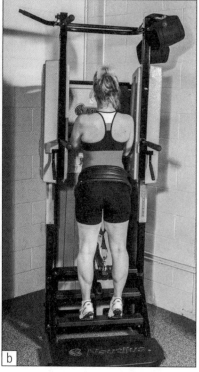

LOW BACK EXTENSION
Erector spinae

Beginning Position

1. Sit all the way back on seat and adjust foot pad so that knees are slightly higher than hips.
2. Secure seat belts across thighs and hips if available.
3. Cross arms on chest.
4. Place upper back firmly against pad with trunk flexed forward.

Backward Movement Phase

1. Push upper back against pad until trunk is fully extended.
2. Keep head in line with torso.
3. Exhale throughout extension movement.

Forward Movement Phase

1. Allow pad to slowly return to starting position.
2. Inhale throughout return movement.

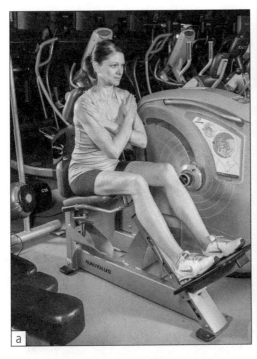
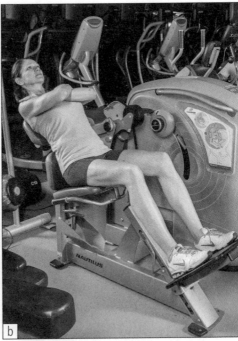

ABDOMINAL FLEXION
Rectus abdominis

Beginning Position

1. Adjust seat so that navel is aligned with machine's axis of rotation.
2. Secure seat belt.
3. Sit with upper back firmly against pad.
4. Place elbows on arm pads and hands on handles.

Forward Movement Phase

1. Pull pad forward slowly by contracting abdominal muscles until trunk is fully flexed (tightening abdominal muscles as much as you can).
2. Keep upper back firmly against pad.
3. Exhale throughout forward movement.

Backward Movement Phase

1. Allow the pad to slowly return to starting position.
2. Inhale throughout return movement.

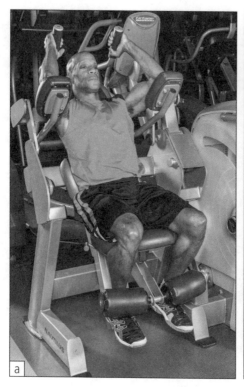
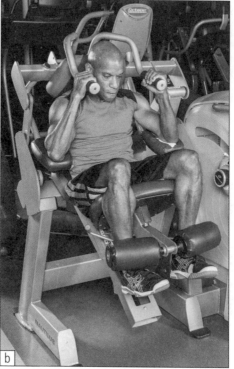

ROTARY TORSO

Rectus abdominis, external obliques, internal obliques

Beginning Position

1. Sit all the way back on seat, facing forward with torso erect.
2. Position left upper arm behind arm pad and right upper arm against (in front of) arm pad.

Rotation Movement Phase

1. Rotate torso slowly to the right about 45 degrees.
2. Exhale throughout rotation.

Return Movement Phase

1. Allow torso to slowly return to starting position (facing forward).
2. Inhale throughout return movement.
3. Change arm position and repeat exercise to the left.

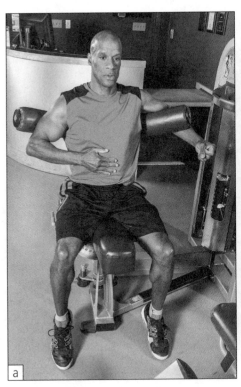 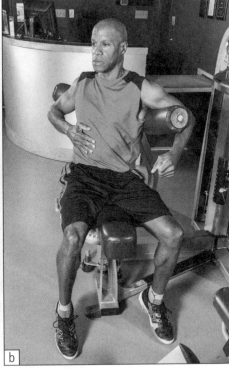

CHEST CROSSOVER
Pectoralis major, anterior deltoids

Beginning Position

1. Adjust seat so that shoulders are in line with machine's axis of rotation and upper arms are parallel to floor.
2. Sit with head, shoulders, and back firmly against seat back.
3. Position forearms against arm pads and hands on handles.

Forward Movement Phase

1. Pull arm pads slowly together, exerting more force with the forearms than with the hands.
2. Keep wrists straight.
3. Exhale throughout pulling movement.

Backward Movement Phase

1. Allow arm pads to slowly return to starting position.
2. Inhale throughout return movement.

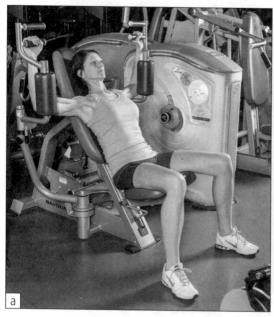
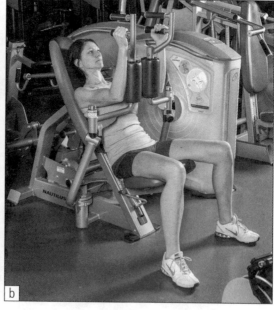

CHEST PRESS
Pectoralis major, anterior deltoids, triceps

Beginning Position
1. Adjust seat so that handles are in line with middle of chest.
2. Sit with head, shoulders, and back against seat back.
3. Grasp handles with palms facing away.

Forward Movement Phase
1. Push handles forward slowly until arms are fully extended.
2. Keep wrists straight.
3. Exhale throughout pushing movement.

Backward Movement Phase
1. Allow handles to return slowly to starting position.
2. Inhale throughout return phase.

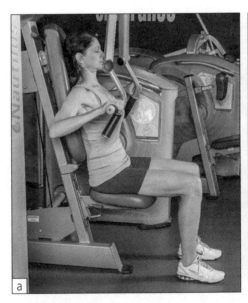 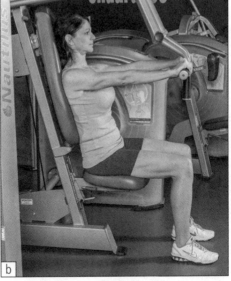

INCLINE PRESS
Pectoralis major, anterior deltoids, triceps

Beginning Position
1. Adjust seat so that handles are below chin level.
2. Sit with head, shoulders, and back against seat pad.
3. Grasp handles with fingers and thumbs, palms facing away.

Upward Movement Phase
1. Push hands upward slowly until arms are fully extended.
2. Keep wrists straight.
3. Exhale throughout pushing movement.

Downward Movement Phase
1. Return handles slowly to starting position.
2. Inhale throughout lowering movement.

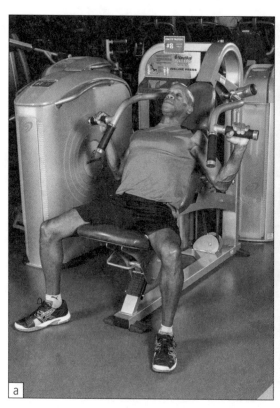
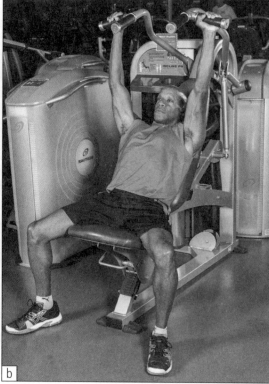

LATERAL RAISE
Deltoids

Beginning Position

1. Adjust seat so that shoulders are in line with machine's axis of rotation.
2. Sit with head, shoulders, and back firmly against seat pad.
3. Position arms against arm pads and hands on handles with arms close to sides.

Upward Movement Phase

1. Lift arm pads upward slowly, exerting more pressure with the arms than with the hands.
2. Keep wrists straight.
3. Stop upward movement when arms are parallel to floor.
4. Exhale throughout lifting movement.

Downward Movement Phase

1. Allow pads to slowly return to starting position.
2. Inhale throughout lowering movement.

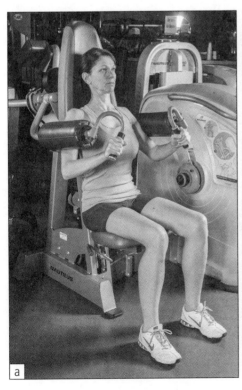 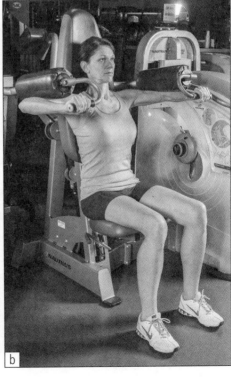

SHOULDER PRESS
Deltoids, triceps, upper trapezius

Beginning Position

1. Adjust seat so that handles are below chin level.
2. Sit with head, shoulders, and back against seat pad.
3. Grasp handles with fingers and thumbs, palms facing away.

Upward Movement Phase

1. Push hands upward slowly until arms are fully extended.
2. Keep wrists straight.
3. Exhale throughout pushing movement.

Downward Movement Phase

1. Return handles slowly to starting position.
2. Inhale throughout lowering movement.

Shoulder Exercise

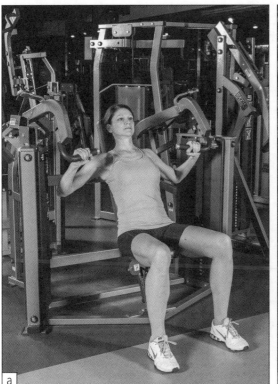

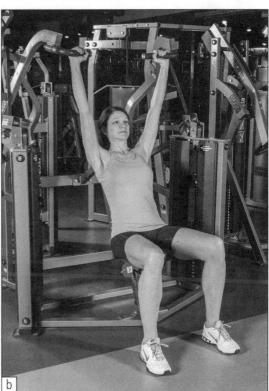

PULLOVER
Latissimus dorsi

Beginning Position

1. Adjust seat so that shoulders are in line with machine's axis of rotation.
2. Sit with back firmly against seat pad, seat belt secured.
3. Place feet on foot lever and press forward to bring arm pads into starting position near face.
4. Position arms against arm pads and hands on bar.
5. Release foot pad.

Downward Movement Phase

1. Pull arm pads downward slowly, leading with elbows until bar touches body.
2. Keep wrists straight.
3. Allow back to round slightly during downward movement.
4. Exhale throughout downward movement.

Upward Movement Phase

1. Allow arm pads to slowly return to starting position.
2. Inhale throughout return movement.

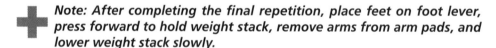 ***Note: After completing the final repetition, place feet on foot lever, press forward to hold weight stack, remove arms from arm pads, and lower weight stack slowly.***

Upper-Back Exercise

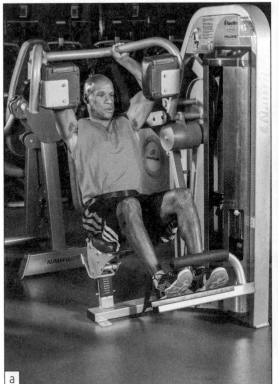 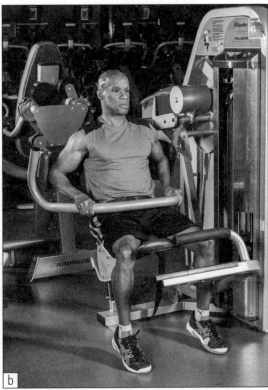

LAT PULLDOWN

Latissimus dorsi, biceps

Beginning Position

1. Place thighs under restraining pads, keeping torso upright.
2. Grip the handles with arms fully extended overhead.

Downward Movement Phase

1. Pull handles downward slowly below chin.
2. Exhale throughout pulling movement.

Upward Movement Phase

1. Return slowly to starting position with arms fully extended.
2. Inhale throughout the upward movement.

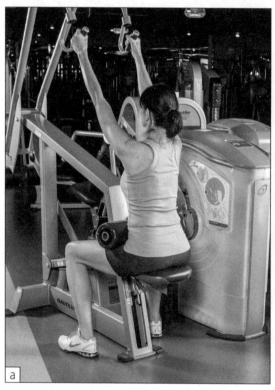
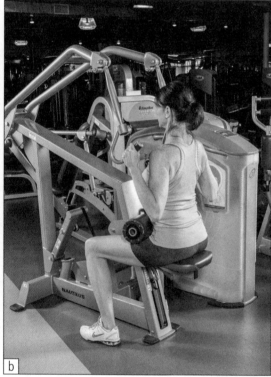

SEATED ROW
Latissimus dorsi, biceps

Beginning Position
1. Adjust seat so that handles are at shoulder level.
2. Sit with chest against chest pad and torso erect.
3. Place feet flat on floor or on foot pad on machine.
4. Grasp each handle with arms fully extended.

Backward Movement Phase
1. Pull handles slowly back toward chest.
2. Keep wrists straight.
3. Exhale throughout pulling movement.

Forward Movement Phase
1. Allow handles to return slowly until arms are fully extended.
2. Inhale throughout return movement.

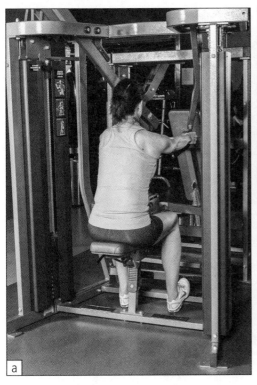
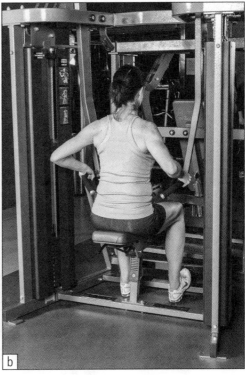

WEIGHT-ASSISTED CHIN-UP
Latissimus dorsi, biceps

Beginning Position
1. Keep in mind that adding weights makes this exercise easier because they counterbalance your body weight.
2. Climb steps and grasp chin-up bar with an underhand grip.
3. Place knees on platform and descend until arms are fully extended.

Upward Movement Phase
1. Pull body upward until chin is above chin-up bar.
2. Keep wrists straight.
3. Keep back straight.
4. Exhale throughout pulling movement.

Downward Movement Phase
1. Return slowly to starting position until arms are fully extended.
2. Inhale throughout return movement.

Upper-Back Exercise

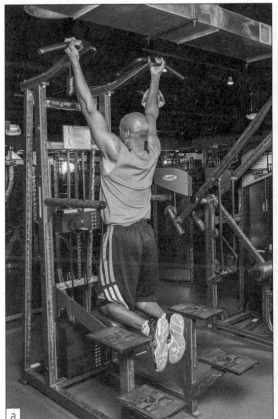 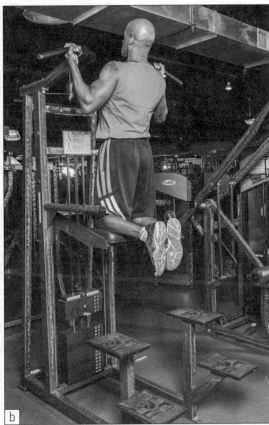

ROWING

Latissimus dorsi, posterior deltoids, rhomboids, middle trapezius

Beginning Position

1. Adjust seat so that upper arms contact center of movement pads when parallel to floor.
2. Sit with head, shoulders, and back against seat pad and feet on foot bar.

Backward Movement Phase

1. Push movement pads backward as far as possible, maintaining an erect torso.
2. Exhale throughout the backward movement phase.

Forward Movement Phase

1. Return movement pads slowly to starting position.
2. Inhale throughout return movement phase.

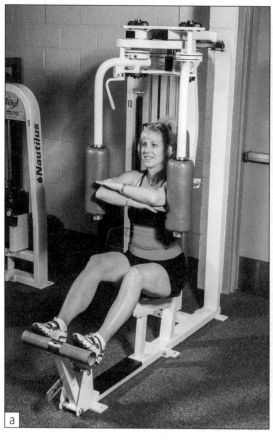
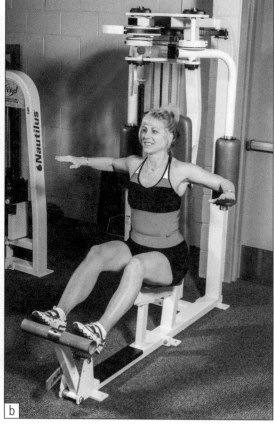

WEIGHT-ASSISTED BAR DIP

Pectoralis major, triceps

Beginning Position

1. Keep in mind that adding weights makes this exercise easier because they counterbalance your body weight.
2. Climb steps and grasp dip bars with hands evenly spaced.
3. Place knees on platform and descend until elbows are flexed about 90 degrees.

Upward Movement Phase

1. Push body upward slowly until arms are fully extended.
2. Keep wrists straight.
3. Keep back straight.
4. Exhale throughout pushing movement.

Downward Movement Phase

1. Return slowly to starting position until elbows are flexed about 90 degrees.
2. Inhale throughout return movement.

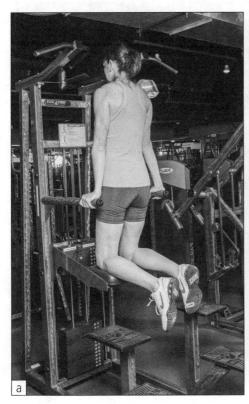
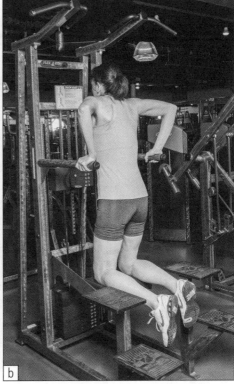

BICEPS CURL
Biceps

Beginning Position
1. Adjust seat so that elbows are in line with machine's axis of rotation and upper arms are angled slightly upward.
2. Grasp handles with underhand grip and with elbows slightly flexed.
3. Sit with head in neutral position and torso erect.

Upward Movement Phase
1. Curl handles upward slowly until elbows are fully flexed.
2. Keep wrists straight.
3. Exhale throughout lifting movement.

Downward Movement Phase
1. Allow handles to return slowly to starting position.
2. Inhale throughout lowering movement.

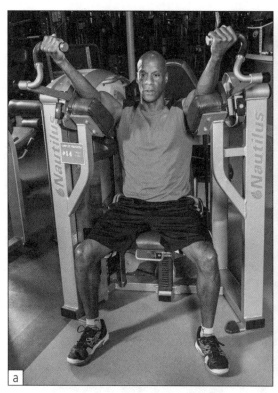 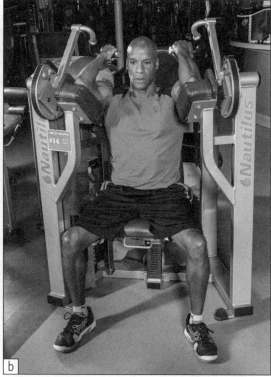

TRICEPS EXTENSION
Triceps

Beginning Position

1. Adjust seat so that elbows are in line with machine's axis of rotation.
2. Sit with back firmly against seat pad.
3. Place sides of hands against hand pads and allow pads to move close to shoulders.

Forward Movement Phase

1. Push handles forward slowly until arms are fully extended.
2. Keep wrists straight.
3. Exhale throughout forward movement.

Backward Movement Phase

1. Allow handles to return slowly to starting position.
2. Inhale throughout return movement.

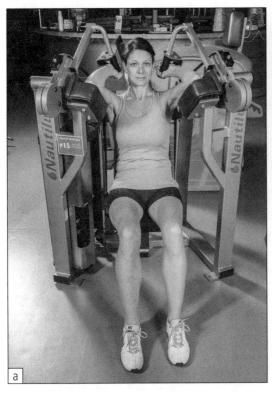
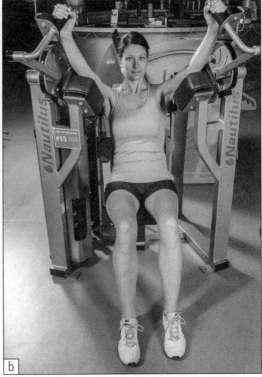

TRICEPS PRESS
Triceps, pectoralis major, anterior deltoids

Beginning Position
1. Adjust seat so that elbows are at 90-degree angles when hands are grasping handles.
2. Sit with erect torso and hands grasping handles directly below shoulders.
3. Secure seat belt.

Downward Movement Phase
1. Push handles downward until arms are fully extended.
2. Keep wrists straight.
3. Exhale throughout pushing movement.

Upward Movement Phase
1. Return handles slowly to starting position.
2. Inhale throughout return movement.

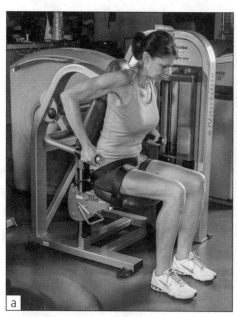
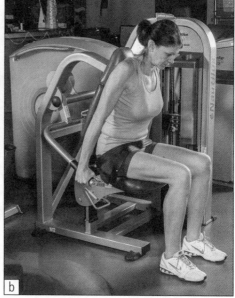

TRICEPS PRESS-DOWN
Triceps

Beginning Position

1. Stand erect with feet hip-width apart and knees slightly flexed.
2. Grasp rope with an overhand grip.
3. Pull rope down until upper arms are perpendicular with floor and touching sides with elbows flexed.

Downward Movement Phase

1. Push rope downward until arms are fully extended.
2. Exhale throughout pushing movement.

Upward Movement Phase

1. Return rope slowly to starting position.
2. Inhale throughout upward movement.

 Note: Prepare for an unexpected upward pull from the rope during the upward movement phase.

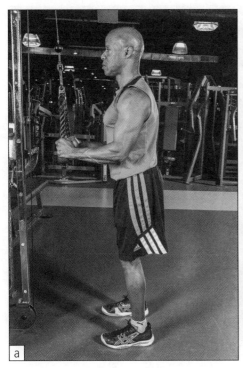 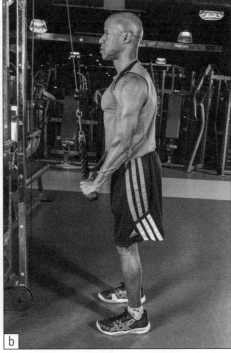

NECK EXTENSION
Neck extensors

Beginning Position

1. Adjust seat so that back of head fits comfortably in head pad.
2. Adjust torso pad for an erect posture.
3. Place back of head against head pad with head angled slightly forward.
4. Grip handles.

Backward Movement Phase

1. Push head pad backward slowly until neck is comfortably extended.
2. Keep torso straight.
3. Exhale throughout backward movement.

Forward Movement Phase

1. Allow head pad to slowly return to starting position with head angled slightly forward.
2. Inhale throughout return movement.

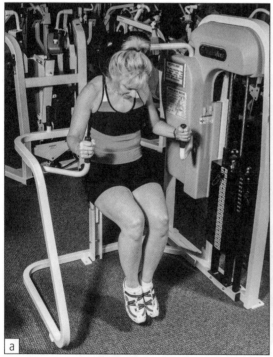
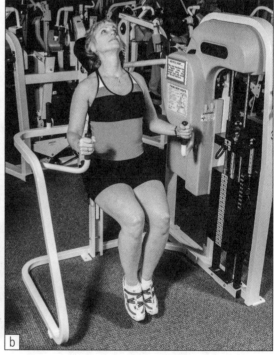

NECK FLEXION
Neck flexors

Beginning Position

1. Adjust seat so that face will fit comfortably against head pad with nose parallel to cross bar.
2. Adjust torso pad for erect posture.
3. Place forehead and cheeks against head pad with head angled slightly backward.
4. Grip handles.

Forward Movement Phase

1. Push head pad forward slowly until the neck is fully flexed.
2. Keep torso straight.
3. Exhale throughout forward movement.

Backward Movement Phase

1. Allow head pad to return slowly to starting position with head angled slightly backward.
2. Inhale throughout return movement.

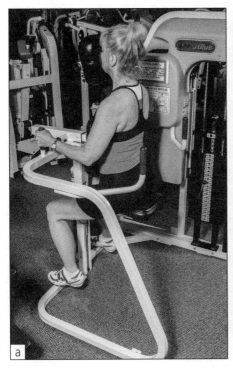 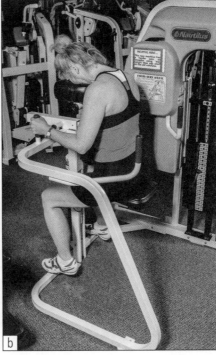

7

Free-Weight Exercises

In chapters 1 to 4 you learned about the many benefits of strength training, how to assess your current strength training status, which training programs in this book are suited to you, keys to training success, and equipment that you will be using. In chapter 5 you learned about grips, stance and body positioning, speed of movement, and breathing techniques, all of which you will apply when performing the 33 barbell, dumbbell, or kettlebell exercises in this chapter. We also identify exercises in which having a spotter is recommended.

As you review the exercises in this chapter and the machine and alternative exercises in chapters 6 and 8, respectively, you will note that some exercises are performed in a rotary movement pattern. That is, the exercise action is circular in nature. Rotary movements, such as leg extension and barbell curl, involve a single-joint action that is typically produced by one or sometimes two major muscle groups. For example, the leg extension exercise addresses the quadriceps muscles and activates the knee joints. Similarly, the barbell curl exercise addresses the biceps muscles and activates the elbow joint.

Other exercises are performed in a linear movement pattern. That is, the exercise action is essentially in a straight line. Linear movements, such as leg press and bench press, involve more than one joint action and are typically produced by two or more major muscle groups. For example, the leg press exercise addresses the quadriceps, hamstrings, and gluteal muscles and activates both the knee and hip joints. Likewise, the bench press exercise addresses the pectoralis major, anterior deltoids, and triceps muscles and activates both the shoulder and elbow joints. We believe that a comprehensive strength training program should include both rotary and linear exercises to maximize overall muscle development.

SQUAT: KETTLEBELLS OR DUMBBELLS
Quadriceps, hamstrings, gluteals

Beginning Position

1. Grasp kettlebells or dumbbells with elbows extended, and stand erect with feet about hip-width apart and parallel to each other.
2. Position kettlebells or dumbbells with palms facing the outside surfaces of thighs.

Downward Movement Phase

1. Keep head up, eyes fixed straight ahead, shoulders back, torso erect, and weight on entire foot throughout the upward and downward movement phases of the exercise.
2. Squat slowly until thighs are parallel to floor.
3. Inhale throughout downward movement phase.

+ *Note: If balance is a problem, try positioning upper back and buttocks against a wall for support (i.e., slide up and down a wall). Do not allow the knees to move farther forward than the toes.*

Upward Movement Phase

1. Begin upward movement by slowly straightening the knees and hips.
2. Exhale throughout upward movement phase.

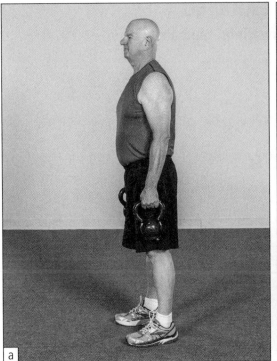

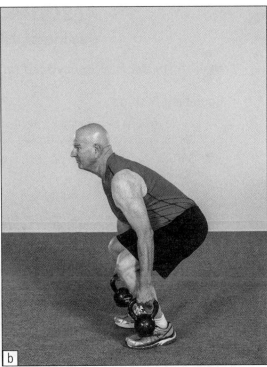

SQUAT: BARBELL

Quadriceps, hamstrings, gluteals

 A spotter is recommended for this exercise.

Beginning Position

1. While the bar is in the rack, position feet shoulder-width apart or wider and grip the bar with palms facing down.
2. Duck under the bar and position bar on shoulders at base of neck, head up, eyes looking ahead.
3. Stand erect to lift bar out of rack.

Downward Movement Phase

1. Keep head up, eyes fixed straight ahead, shoulders back, torso erect, and weight on entire foot throughout the upward and downward movement phases of the exercise.
2. Squat slowly until thighs are parallel to floor.
3. Inhale throughout downward movement phase.

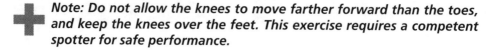 *Note: Do not allow the knees to move farther forward than the toes, and keep the knees over the feet. This exercise requires a competent spotter for safe performance.*

Upward Movement Phase

1. Begin upward movement by slowly straightening knees and hips.
2. Exhale throughout upward movement phase.
3. Return bar to rack carefully after completing the set.

Leg Exercise

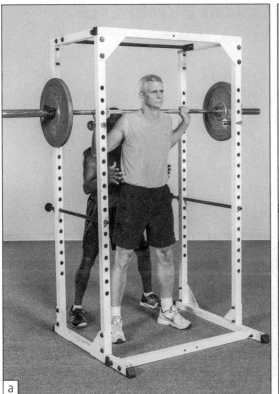 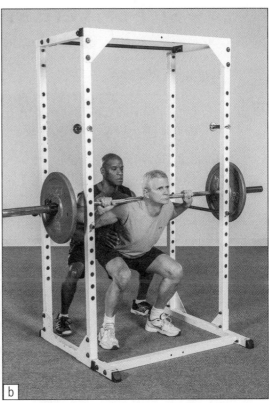

STEP-UP: KETTLEBELLS OR DUMBBELLS
Quadriceps, hamstrings, gluteals

Beginning Position

1. While in front of step or bench, grasp kettlebells or dumbbells with palms facing outer thighs and elbows extended, then stand erect with feet about hip-width apart and parallel to each other.

Upward Movement Phase

1. Keep head up, eyes fixed straight ahead, shoulders back, and torso erect throughout the exercise.
2. Place right foot on step, followed by the left foot, so you are standing on step.
3. Exhale throughout upward movement phase.

Downward Movement Phase

1. Place right foot on the floor, followed by left foot, so you are standing on floor.
2. Inhale throughout downward movement phase.

Note: Alternate the lead foot every repetition.

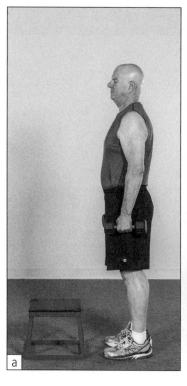
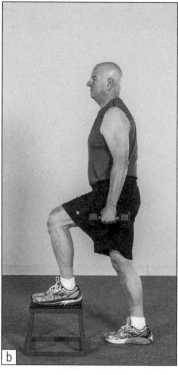
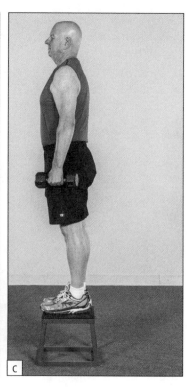

a   b   c

LUNGE: KETTLEBELLS OR DUMBBELLS
Quadriceps, hamstrings, gluteals

Beginning Position

1. Grasp kettlebells or dumbbells with palms facing outer thighs, elbows extended, and stand erect with feet about hip-width apart and parallel to each other.

Forward Movement Phase

1. Keep head up, eyes fixed straight ahead, shoulders back, and torso erect throughout exercise.
2. Take a long step forward with right foot and bend right knee to a 90-degree angle.
3. Step forward far enough that the right knee is directly above (not in front of) right foot.
4. Inhale throughout forward movement phase.

Backward Movement Phase

1. Push off right foot and return to standing position with feet parallel to each other.
2. Exhale throughout backward movement phase.

Note: Alternate the lead foot every repetition.

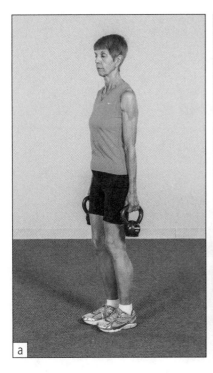
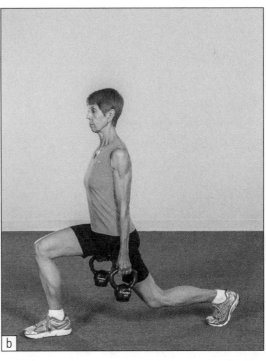

HEEL RAISE: KETTLEBELLS OR DUMBBELLS

Gastrocnemius, soleus

Beginning Position

1. Grasp kettlebells or dumbbells with palms facing outside of thighs, elbows extended, and stand erect.
2. Position kettlebells or dumbbells alongside outside surfaces of thighs.
3. Place balls of feet on a stable, elevated surface (approximately 1 to 2 inches, or 2.5 to 5 cm high) with feet hip-width apart and parallel to each other.

Upward Movement Phase

1. Keep head up, eyes fixed straight ahead, shoulders back, torso erect, and weight on balls of feet throughout upward and downward movement phases of exercise.
2. Rise slowly on toes while keeping torso erect and knees straight.
3. Exhale throughout upward movement phase.

Downward Movement Phase

1. Lower heels as far as comfortable while keeping torso erect and knees straight.
2. Inhale throughout lowering movement phase.

Leg Exercise

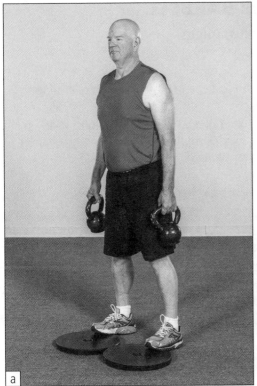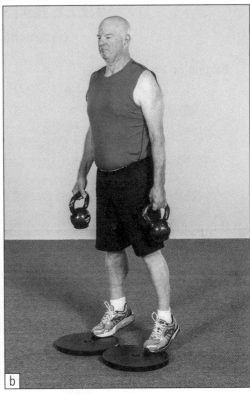

HEEL RAISE: BARBELL
Gastrocnemius, soleus

Beginning Position

1. Stand erect, position feet shoulder-width apart, and grasp bar with palms facing forward.
2. Hold bar against thighs using an alternated grip with elbows straight, head up, and eyes looking ahead. (Another way to perform this exercise is with the bar on shoulders at base of neck. Note that this variation requires a spotter.)
3. Place balls of feet on a stable, elevated surface (approximately 1 to 2 inches, or 2.5 to 5 cm high) with feet hip-width apart and parallel to each other.

Upward Movement Phase

1. Keep head up, eyes fixed straight ahead, shoulders back, torso erect, and weight on balls of feet throughout upward and downward movement phases of exercise.
2. Rise on toes slowly while keeping torso erect and knees straight.
3. Exhale throughout upward movement phase.

Downward Movement Phase

1. Lower heels as far as comfortable while keeping torso erect and knees straight.
2. Inhale throughout lowering movement phase.

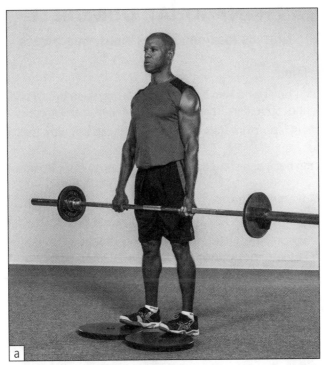

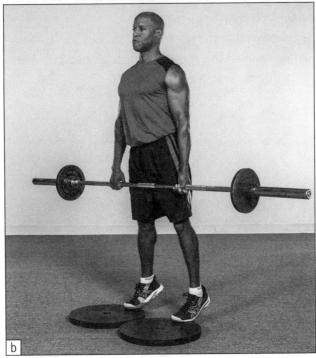

FRONT SQUAT: DUMBBELL
Gluteus maximus, hamstrings, quadriceps

Beginning Position

1. Grasp a dumbbell with two hands (palms facing each other) and position dumbbell in front of shoulders, midchest location, and stand erect.
2. Position feet approximately shoulder-width apart with toes pointed slightly outward.
3. Slightly arch back and shoulders with chest out so back is flat and torso is erect.

Downward Movement Phase

1. Allow hips and knees to flex at the same rate and keep torso erect and back flat.
2. Do not lean forward while squatting; keep shoulders back and chest out with dumbbell in the same position at front of shoulders.
3. Keep heels in full contact with the floor and knees aligned over feet.
4. Continue the downward movement until thighs are parallel to the floor. If heels lift off the floor or you begin to lean forward, you squatted down too far; perform remaining repetitions with a shallower squat.
5. Inhale during this movement phase.

Upward Movement Phase

1. Extend hips and knees at the same rate to stand back up to the initial position.
2. Keep back flat, heels on the floor, and knees aligned over feet.
3. Exhale during this movement phase.

Leg Exercise

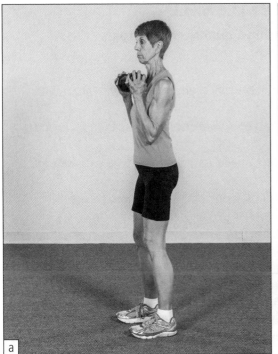 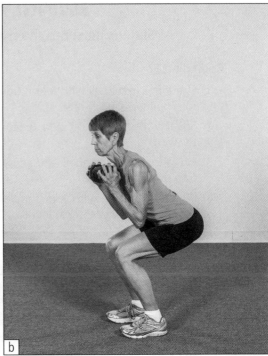

SWING: KETTLEBELL
Gluteus maximus, hamstrings, quadriceps, deltoids

Beginning Position

1. Straddle a kettlebell with feet moderately wider than shoulder-width apart with toes pointed slightly outward.
2. Squat with torso erect and grasp kettlebell with both hands, thumbs facing forward.
3. Stand up with kettlebell and allow it to hang between your legs with elbows fully extended.
4. Slightly arch back with your shoulders back and chest out so torso is erect and shoulders are over the kettlebell.

Forward and Upward Movement

1. To cause the kettlebell to start moving, squat and use a small effort of your arms to move the kettlebell back between legs. (For the rest of the exercise, arms do not play an active role in moving the kettlebell.)
2. At the bottom of the swing, forearms (with your elbows fully extended) are pressed against inner thighs, and the kettlebell is behind you.
3. To move the kettlebell forward and up, thrust your hips forward and upward.
4. Keep shoulders back and chest out.
5. Guide kettlebell up with elbows still fully extended until kettlebell reaches approximately chest or shoulder height.
6. Exhale during this movement phase.

Backward and Downward Movement

1. After kettlebell reaches highest position, lower it under control to its lowest position with elbows straight.
2. As the kettlebell moves downward to the bottom of the swing, squat slightly with hips and shoulders back, chest out, and forearms pressed against inner thighs.
3. To complete set, allow kettlebell to swing forward, but do not extend hips and knees to continue swing.
4. Once swing has stopped, place kettlebell on floor between feet.
5. Inhale during this movement phase.

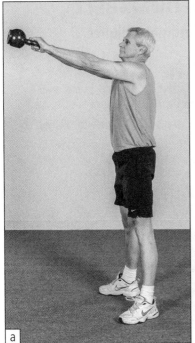
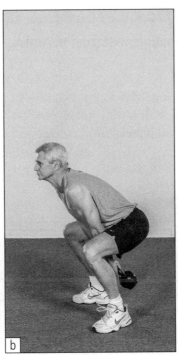
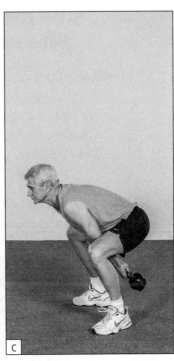

SIDE BEND: KETTLEBELL OR DUMBBELL
Rectus abdominis, external obliques, internal obliques

Beginning Position

1. Grasp kettlebell or dumbbell in right hand with arm extended and stand erect with feet about hip-width apart and parallel to each other.
2. Position kettlebell or dumbbell with palm facing the outside surface of right thigh.
3. Keep shoulders square with hips and arms straight throughout the exercise. Do not bend forward or backward.

Upward Movement Phase

1. Lift kettlebell or dumbbell upward by bending at waist to the left.
2. Exhale throughout upward movement phase.

Downward Movement Phase

1. Lower kettlebell or dumbbell downward as far as possible by bending at waist to the right.
2. Inhale throughout downward movement phase.

Note: After completing all of the repetitions with the kettlebell or dumbbell in the right hand, switch the kettlebell or dumbbell to the left hand and repeat.

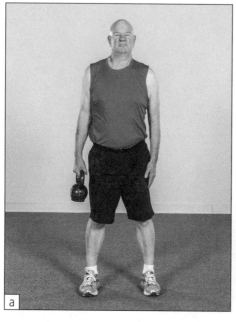
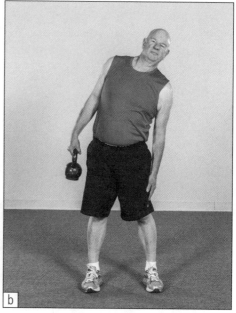

DEADLIFT: KETTLEBELLS OR DUMBBELLS

Erector spinae, quadriceps, hamstrings, gluteals

Beginning Position

1. Assume the starting lifting position described in chapter 5.
2. Position kettlebells or dumbbells in hands with palms facing outside surfaces of ankles and elbows extended.

Upward Movement Phase

1. Lift kettlebells or dumbbells off the floor by extending hips while keeping elbows straight and back flat as described in chapter 5.
2. Once kettlebells or dumbbells are above knees, move hips forward.
3. Continue to extend hips and knees until body reaches a fully erect position.
4. Exhale through this movement phase.

Downward Movement Phase

1. Allow hips and knees to flex to slowly lower kettlebells or dumbbells to the floor.
2. Maintain a flat back position.
3. Inhale through this movement phase.

Note: Your back should remain in a relatively stable position throughout the exercise. Most of the movement is around the hip and knee joints.

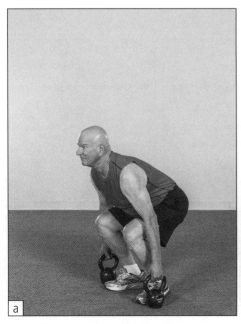
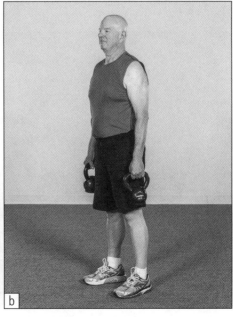

DEADLIFT: BARBELL
Erector spinae, quadriceps, hamstrings, gluteals

Beginning Position

1. Assume starting lifting position described in chapter 5.
2. Place hands on bar slightly wider than shoulder-width apart and with elbows extended.
3. Place feet flat on floor with the bar 1 inch (3 cm) in front of the shins and over balls of feet.

Upward Movement Phase

1. Lift bar off floor by extending hips while keeping elbows extended and back flat as described in chapter 5.
2. Keep bar close to shins until bar reaches a point above knees.
3. Once bar is above knees, move hips forward to move thighs against and under knees under bar.
4. Continue to extend hips and knees until body reaches a fully erect position.
5. Exhale through this movement phase.

Downward Movement Phase

1. Allow hips and knees to flex to slowly lower bar to floor.
2. Maintain a flat back position; do not flex torso forward.
3. Inhale through this movement phase.

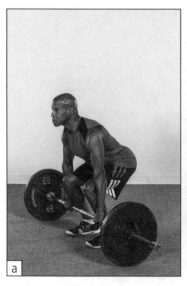
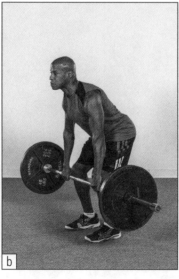
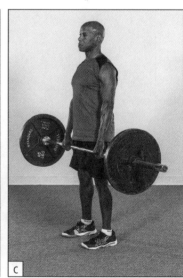

a   b   c

CHEST FLY: DUMBBELLS
Pectoralis major, anterior deltoids

 A spotter is recommended for this exercise.

Beginning Position

1. Lie faceup on bench with legs straddling it and knees flexed at 90 degrees, feet flat on floor.
2. Grasp dumbbells palms facing up, elbows slightly flexed.
3. Keep head, shoulders, and buttocks in contact with the bench and feet in contact with the floor throughout the exercise.
4. Push dumbbells in unison to a position over chest with elbows slightly flexed.

Downward Movement Phase

1. Lower dumbbells slowly and in unison, keeping elbows slightly flexed and perpendicular to torso until upper arms are parallel to floor.
2. Inhale throughout lowering movement phase.

Upward Movement Phase

1. Lift dumbbells upward in unison to starting position with elbows slightly flexed.
2. Exhale throughout upward movement phase.

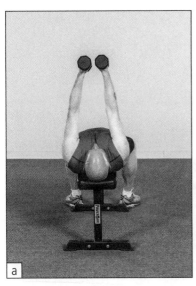
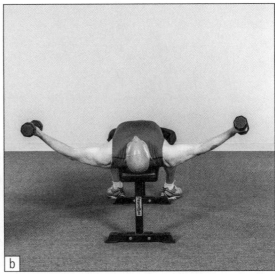

BENCH PRESS: DUMBBELLS
Pectoralis major, anterior deltoids, triceps

 A spotter is recommended for this exercise.

Beginning Position

1. Lie on back with legs straddling bench, knees flexed at 90 degrees, feet flat on floor.
2. Grasp dumbbells so palms face forward and push upward until arms are fully extended above chest.
3. Keep head, shoulders, and buttocks in contact with the bench and feet in contact with the floor throughout the exercise.

Downward Movement Phase

1. Lower dumbbells slowly and evenly to chest.
2. Inhale throughout lowering movement phase.

Upward Movement Phase

1. Press dumbbells upward in unison until arms are fully extended.
2. Exhale throughout upward movement phase.

Chest Exercise

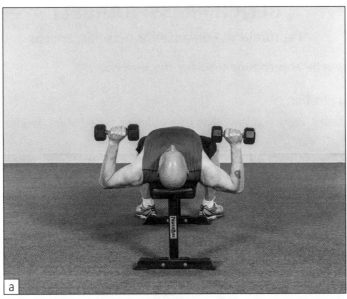

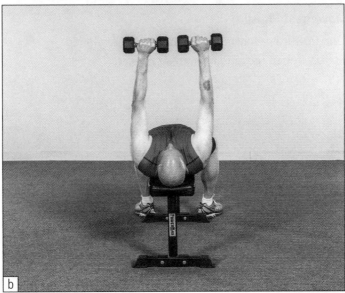

BENCH PRESS: BARBELL

Pectoralis major, anterior deltoids, triceps

 A spotter is recommended for this exercise.

Beginning Position

1. Lie on back with legs straddling bench, knees flexed at 90 degrees, feet flat on floor.
2. Grasp barbell with palms facing upward and slightly wider than shoulders and then push upward until elbows are fully extended above chest.
3. Keep head, shoulders, and buttocks in contact with bench and feet in contact with the floor throughout the exercise.

Downward Movement Phase

1. Lower bar slowly and evenly to chest.
2. Inhale throughout the lowering movement phase.

Upward Movement Phase

1. Press bar upward evenly until elbows are fully extended.
2. Exhale throughout pressing movement phase.

Chest Exercise

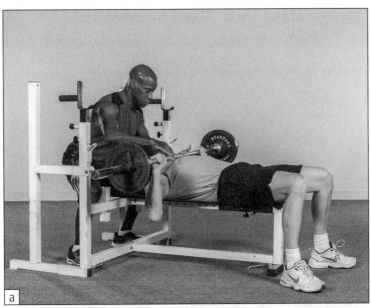

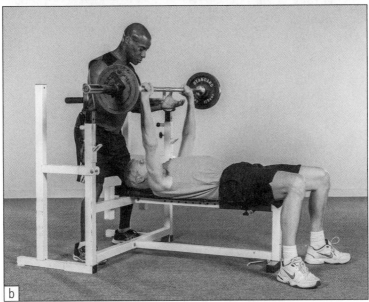

INCLINE PRESS: BARBELL

Pectoralis major, anterior deltoids, triceps

 A spotter is recommended for this exercise.

Beginning Position

1. Sit with head, shoulders, and back in contact with incline bench and feet flat on floor throughout exercise.
2. Grasp barbell with palms facing forward slightly wider than shoulders; push upward until elbows are fully extended above shoulders.

Downward Movement Phase

1. Lower bar slowly and evenly to shoulder level.
2. Inhale throughout lowering movement phase.

Upward Movement Phase

1. Press bar upward evenly until elbows are fully extended above shoulders.
2. Exhale throughout pressing movement phase.

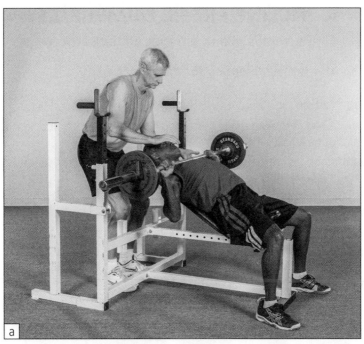

a

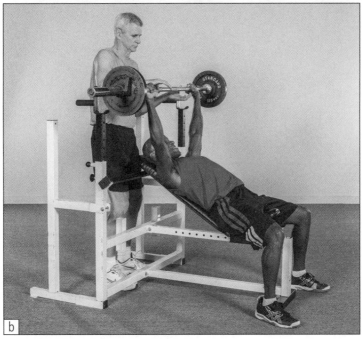

b

INCLINE PRESS: DUMBBELLS
Pectoralis major, anterior deltoids, triceps

 A spotter is recommended for this exercise.

Beginning Position

1. Sit with head, shoulders, and back against incline bench and feet flat on floor throughout exercise.
2. Grasp dumbbells with palms facing forward and positioned directly above shoulders with elbows fully extended.

Downward Movement Phase

1. Lower dumbbells slowly and evenly to shoulder level.
2. Inhale throughout lowering movement phase.

Upward Movement Phase

1. Press dumbbells upward evenly until elbows are fully extended above shoulders.
2. Exhale throughout pressing movement phase.

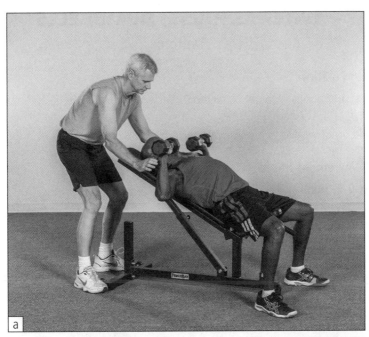

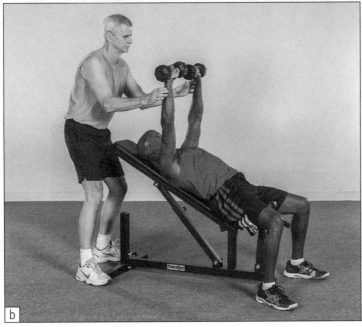

LATERAL RAISE: DUMBBELLS
Deltoids

Beginning Position

1. Grasp dumbbells with palms facing outside surfaces of thighs and elbows slightly flexed.
2. Stand erect with feet hip-width apart.

Upward Movement Phase

1. Slowly lift dumbbells upward, palms facing downward, in unison until they reach shoulder level (parallel to floor).
2. Exhale throughout the upward movement phase.

Downward Movement Phase

1. Slowly lower dumbbells in unison to starting position.
2. Inhale throughout lowering movement phase.

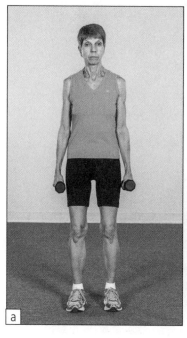
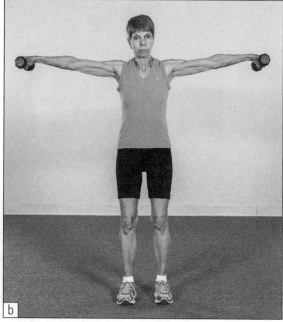

SEATED PRESS: DUMBBELLS

Deltoids, triceps, upper trapezius

 A spotter is recommended for this exercise.

Beginning Position

1. Grasp dumbbells with palms facing forward and position at shoulder height.
2. Sit with legs straddling bench and feet in contact with floor at all times.

Note: If you're using an upright or adjustable bench, keep head and entire back in contact with the bench.

Upward Movement Phase

1. Slowly push dumbbells upward in unison until elbows are fully extended over shoulders.
2. Exhale throughout pushing movement phase.

Downward Movement Phase

1. Slowly lower dumbbells in unison to shoulder level.
2. Inhale throughout lowering movement phase.

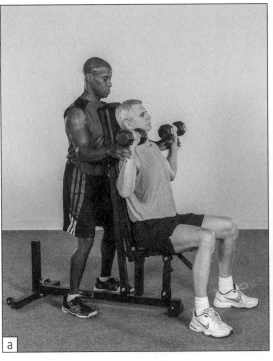
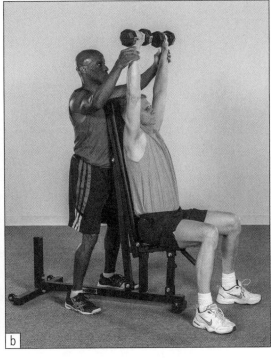

ALTERNATING SHOULDER PRESS: DUMBBELLS
Deltoids, triceps, upper trapezius

Beginning Position

1. Grasp dumbbells with palms facing forward positioned just above shoulder level.
2. Stand with feet about shoulder-width apart and with torso erect.

Upward and Downward Movement Phases

1. Slowly extend left elbow overhead without moving right arm and exhale during the overhead movement.
2. Slowly lower left arm to starting position while inhaling.
3. Slowly extend right elbow overhead without moving left arm and while exhaling.
4. Slowly lower right arm to starting position and while inhaling.
5. Continue alternating right and left arm pressing movements, exhaling and inhaling as previously described.

Note: Maintain erect posture throughout the dumbbell alternating shoulder press exercise, making certain not to lean backward at any time.

Shoulder Exercise

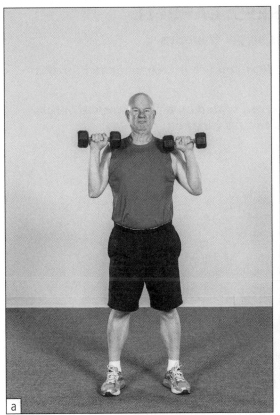 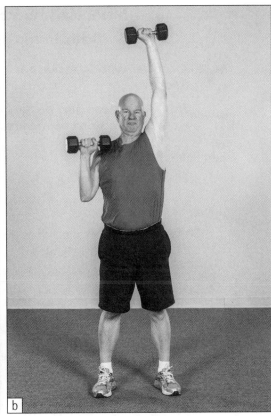

STANDING PRESS: BARBELL

Deltoids, triceps, upper trapezius

 A spotter who is at least as tall as you are is recommended for this exercise.

This exercise can also be performed seated on a flat or incline bench. A spotter is also recommended for this variation.

Beginning Position

1. Follow the guidelines in chapter 5 for lifting the weight off floor to the shoulders.

Upward Movement Phase

1. Tilt head slightly backward while pushing bar straight up (just missing your chin) until elbows are fully extended.
2. Keep wrists straight and directly above elbows.
3. Do not tilt head too far back or lean backward as the bar is pressed overhead.
4. Exhale during this movement phase.

Downward Movement Phase

1. Allow elbows to flex to lower bar to initial position.
2. Tilt head slightly so bar does not hit the head, nose, or chin.
3. Keep wrists straight and directly above elbows.
4. After the last repetition, place the bar on the floor using guidelines for lowering a weight discussed in chapter 5.
5. Inhale during this movement phase.

Shoulder Exercise

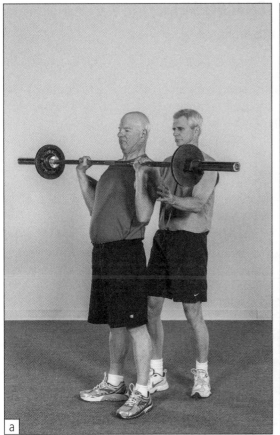

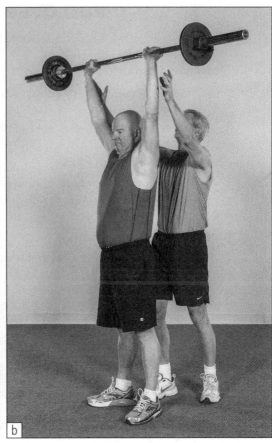

PULLOVER: DUMBBELL
Latissimus dorsi

Beginning Position

1. Grasp dumbbell with both hands (palms facing each other) and move to position behind head.
2. Lie faceup on bench with feet flat on floor.

Downward Movement Phase

1. Lower dumbbell slowly to starting position.
2. Inhale throughout lowering movement phase.

Upward Movement Phase

1. Lift (pull) dumbbell upward and forward until it is just above chest.
2. Exhale throughout upward movement phase.

Note: Keep elbows flexed and close to head throughout the exercise.

Upper-Back Exercise

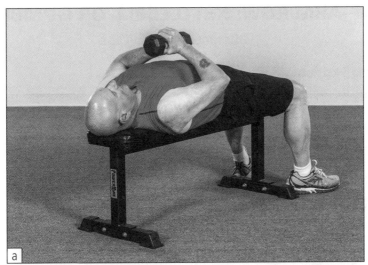

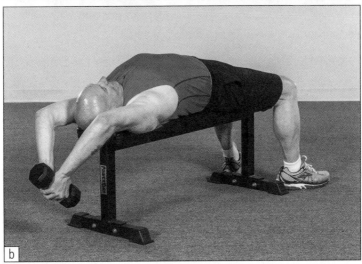

ONE-ARM ROW: KETTLEBELL OR DUMBBELL
Latissimus dorsi, biceps

Beginning Position

1. Grasp the kettlebell or dumbbell with right hand and support weight by placing left hand and knee on the bench, keeping right leg straight and right foot flat on floor.
2. Position kettlebell or dumbbell so that palm faces bench, keeping elbow straight.
3. Keep back flat throughout exercise.

Upward Movement Phase

1. Slowly pull kettlebell or dumbbell to chest height.
2. Exhale throughout pulling movement phase.

Downward Movement Phase

1. Slowly lower kettlebell or dumbbell to starting position.
2. Inhale throughout lowering movement phase.

Note: Repeat exercise from beginning position with left arm and reversed leg positions.

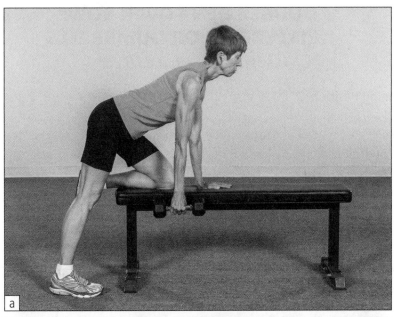

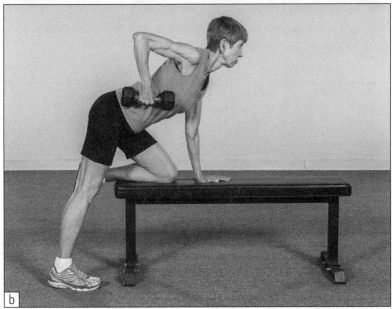

DOUBLE BENT-OVER ROW: KETTLEBELLS OR DUMBBELLS

Latissimus dorsi, rhomboids

Beginning Position

1. Grasp kettlebells so that palms face each other and then assume a slightly flexed knee position with the upper body positioned slightly above parallel to the floor.
2. Upper back should be flat and rigid, not rounded or hunched over.
3. Maintain this knee and torso position throughout the exercise.
4. Allow kettlebells to hang straight down with elbows fully extended.

Upward Movement Phase

1. Pull kettlebells up to lower chest or the upper part of abdomen.
2. Keep wrists straight.
3. Exhale during this movement phase.

Downward Movement Phase

1. Allow elbows to extend to lower kettlebells back to initial position.
2. Inhale while lowering kettlebells.

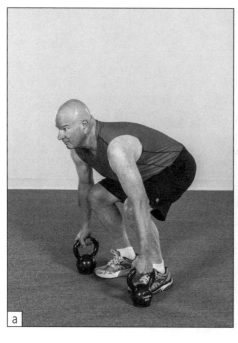 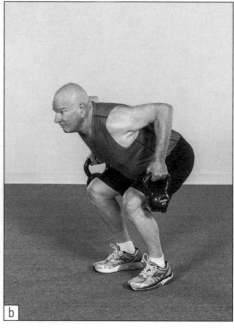

REVERSE FLY: DUMBBELLS

Latissimus dorsi, trapezius, rhomboids, upper trapezius

Beginning Position

1. Flex knees about a quarter of the way and flex torso forward so that it is slightly above parallel to floor. Upper back should be flat and rigid, not rounded or hunched over. Maintain this knee and torso position throughout exercise.
2. Grasp dumbbells with palms facing down.

Upward Movement Phase

1. While keeping elbows and wrists straight and palms facing downward, lift or pull dumbbells upward until parallel to floor.
2. Exhale through upward movement.

Downward Movement Phase

1. Lower dumbbells to the starting position.
2. Inhale through this movement phase.

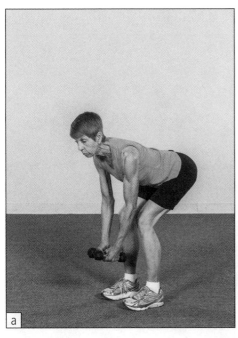 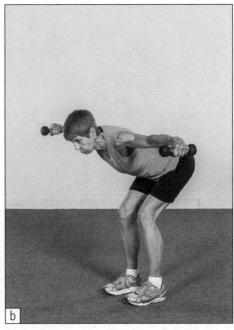

STANDING BICEPS CURL: BARBELL
Biceps

Beginning Position

1. Grasp barbell with an underhand or palms facing up grip, elbow straight. Ensure that upper arms remain perpendicular to floor and held against sides throughout exercise.
2. Stand erect with feet hip-width apart and parallel to each other.

Upward Movement Phase

1. Slowly curl barbell upward toward shoulders until palms face chest.
2. Exhale throughout curling phase.

Downward Movement Phase

1. Slowly lower barbell until elbows are fully extended.
2. Inhale throughout lowering movement phase.

Note: Make sure the upper arms remain perpendicular to floor and against sides throughout this exercise.

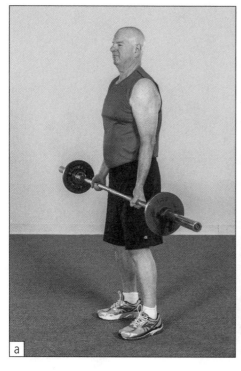 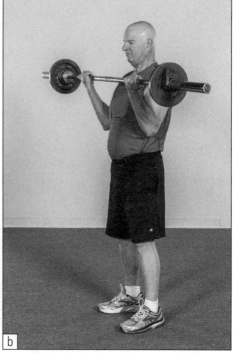

STANDING BICEPS CURL: DUMBBELLS
Biceps

Beginning Position

1. Grasp dumbbells with an underhand grip, elbows straight. Ensure that upper arms remain perpendicular to floor and held against sides throughout exercise.
2. Stand erect with feet about hip-width apart and parallel to each other.

Upward Movement Phase

1. Slowly curl dumbbells upward in unison toward shoulders until palms face the chest.
2. Exhale throughout upward movement phase.

Downward Movement Phase

1. Slowly lower dumbbells in unison to starting position.
2. Inhale throughout lowering movement phase.

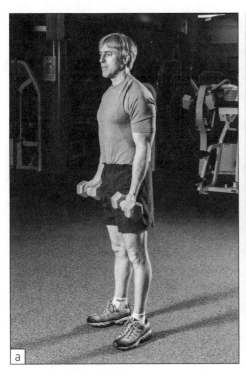 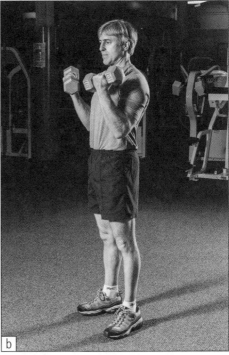

INCLINE CURL: DUMBBELLS
Biceps

Beginning Position

1. Sit on an incline bench with shoulders and back against seat pad and feet on floor.
2. Grasp dumbbells with palms facing forward, elbows straight, and arms perpendicular to floor.

Upward Movement Phase

1. Slowly curl dumbbells upward until palms face chest.
2. Exhale throughout upward movement phase.

Downward Movement Phase

1. Slowly lower dumbbells to starting position.
2. Inhale throughout lowering movement phase.

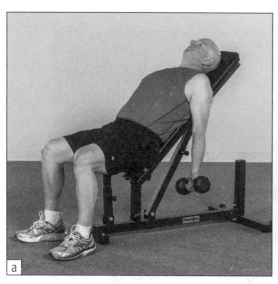

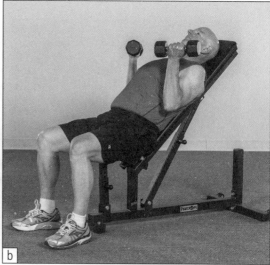

PREACHER CURL: DUMBBELLS
Biceps

Beginning Position

1. Sit on preacher bench with upper arms supported on diagonal arm pad and with feet on floor.
2. Grasp dumbbells with palms facing up and elbows nearly extended.

Upward Movement Phase

1. Slowly curl dumbbells upward until palms face chest.
2. Exhale throughout upward movement phase.

Downward Movement Phase

1. Slowly lower dumbbells to starting position.
2. Inhale throughout lowering movement phase.

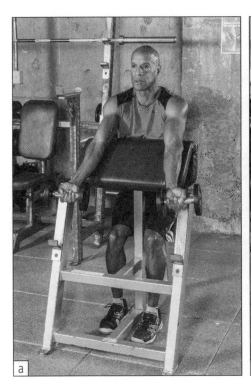

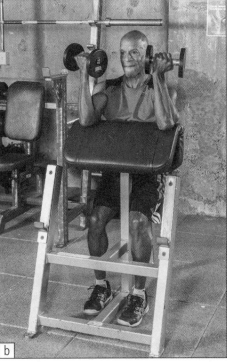

CONCENTRATION CURL: DUMBBELL
Biceps

Beginning Position

1. Sit on bench and grasp dumbbell in left hand with left elbow braced against left thigh. Feet should be shoulder-width apart and upper body should lean slightly forward. Left elbow should remain firmly braced against thigh throughout the exercise.
2. Begin with left elbow bent and palm facing forward.

Upward Movement Phase

1. Slowly curl dumbbell toward chin.
2. Exhale throughout curling movement phase.

Downward Movement Phase

1. Slowly lower dumbbell back to starting position.
2. Inhale throughout lowering movement phase.
3. Repeat from beginning position with right arm (right elbow on right thigh).

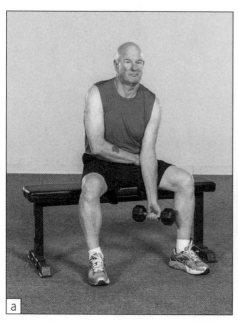
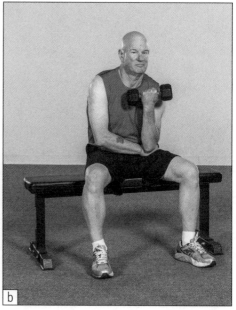

OVERHEAD TRICEPS EXTENSION: DUMBBELL

Triceps

 A spotter is recommended for this exercise.

Beginning Position

1. Grasp one dumbbell with both hands, palms facing each other, and stand erect with feet about hip-width apart.
2. Lift dumbbell upward until elbows are fully extended directly above head.
3. Keep upper arms perpendicular to floor throughout exercise.

Downward Movement Phase

1. Slowly lower dumbbell toward base of neck.
2. Inhale throughout lowering movement phase.

Upward Movement Phase

1. Slowly lift dumbbell upward until elbows are fully extended.
2. Exhale throughout lifting movement phase.

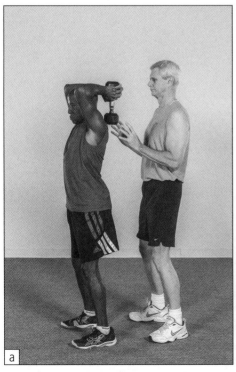

a

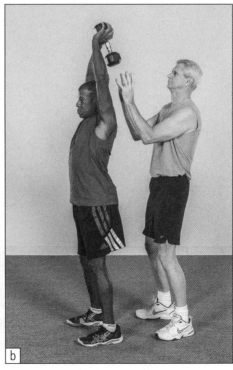

b

LYING TRICEPS EXTENSION: DUMBBELLS

Triceps

 A spotter is recommended for this exercise.

Beginning Position

1. Lie faceup on flat bench with feet on floor.
2. Grasp dumbbells with palms facing each other.
3. Lift dumbbells upward until elbows are fully extended directly above shoulders.

Note: Keep upper arms perpendicular to floor and inside of upper arms next to ears throughout exercise.

Downward Movement Phase

1. Slowly lower dumbbells until they are near the forehead.
2. Inhale throughout lowering movement phase.

Upward Movement Phase

1. Slowly push dumbbells upward until elbows are fully extended above shoulders.
2. Exhale throughout upward movement phase.

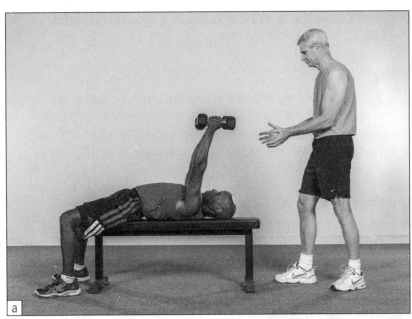

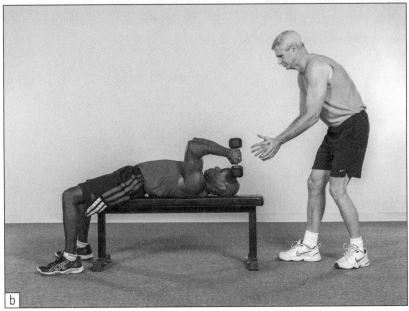

TRICEPS KICKBACK: DUMBBELL
Triceps

Beginning Position

1. Grasp dumbbell with right hand and support weight by placing left hand and knee on bench, keeping the right leg straight and right foot flat on floor.
2. Position dumbbell so that palm faces bench.
3. Lift dumbbell up with right hand and flex the elbow 90 degrees while keeping upper arm close to ribs.

Upward Movement Phase

1. Extend right elbow until it is straight and parallel to floor.
2. Keep upper part of right arm against torso.
3. Keep right wrist straight and body stationary.
4. Exhale through this movement phase.

Downward Movement Phase

1. Allow the right elbow to flex to move the dumbbell to starting position.
2. Inhale through this movement phase.

Back-of-Arm Exercise

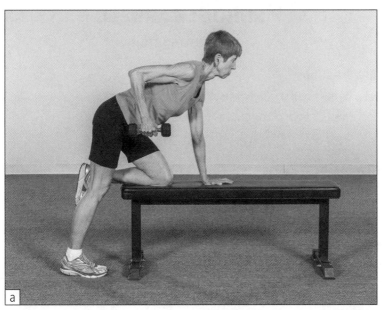

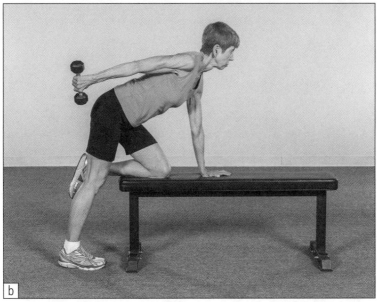

SHRUG: BARBELL
Upper trapezius

Beginning Position

1. Grasp barbell with palms facing body, arms at sides and elbows fully extended.
2. Keep arms straight throughout the exercise.
3. Stand erect with feet hip-width apart.

Upward Movement Phase

1. Elevate (shrug) the shoulders toward ears as high as possible.
2. Exhale throughout shrugging movement phase.

Downward Movement Phase

1. Slowly lower barbell to starting position.
2. Exhale throughout shrugging movement phase.

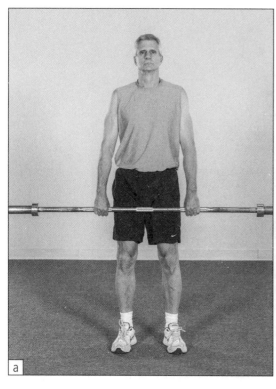
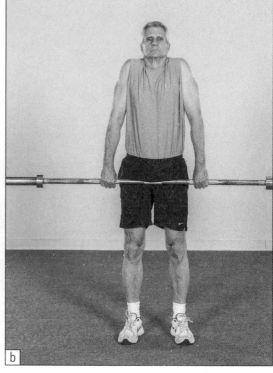

SHRUG: DUMBBELLS OR KETTLEBELLS
Upper trapezius

Beginning Position

1. Grasp kettlebells or dumbbells with palms facing thighs, arms at sides, and elbows fully extended. Keep arms straight throughout exercise.
2. Stand erect with feet hip-width apart.

Upward Movement Phase

1. Elevate (shrug) shoulders in unison toward ears as high as possible.
2. Exhale throughout shrugging movement phase.

Downward Movement Phase

1. Slowly lower kettlebells or dumbbells in unison to starting position.
2. Inhale throughout lowering movement phase.

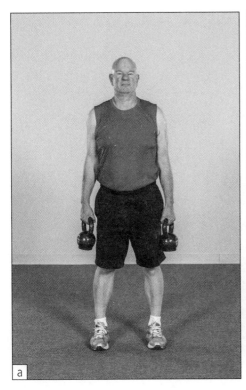
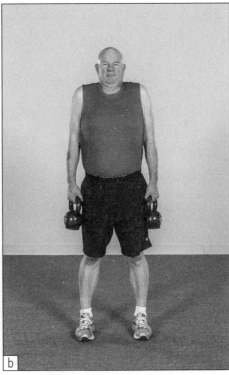

a   b

8

Alternative-Equipment Exercises

In chapters 1 to 4 you learned about the many benefits of strength training, how to assess your current strength training status, which training programs in this book are suited to you, keys to training success, and equipment that you will be using. In chapter 5 you learned about grips, stance and body positioning, speed of movement, and breathing techniques, all of which you will apply when performing the 23 resistance band, exercise ball, or body-weight exercises in this chapter. Refer to the discussion in chapter 4 regarding selecting the correct size of the ball and thickness of resistance bands for the exercises described in this chapter.

As you review the alternative exercises in this chapter and the machine and free-weight exercises in chapters 6 and 7, you will note that some exercises are performed in a rotary movement pattern. That is, the exercise action is circular in nature. Rotary movements, such as leg extension and barbell curl, involve a single-joint action that is typically produced by one or sometimes two major muscle groups. For example, the leg extension exercise addresses the quadriceps muscles and activates the knee joints. Similarly, the barbell curl exercise addresses the biceps muscles and activates the elbow joints.

Other exercises are performed in a linear movement pattern. That is, the exercise action is essentially in a straight line. Linear movements, such as leg press and bench press, involve more than one joint action and are typically produced by two or more major muscle groups. For example, the leg press exercise addresses the quadriceps, hamstring, and gluteal muscles and activates both the knee and hip joints. Likewise, the bench press exercise addresses the pectoralis major, anterior deltoid, and triceps muscles and activates both the shoulder and elbow joints. We believe that a comprehensive strength training program should include both rotary and linear exercises to maximize overall muscular development.

WALL SQUAT:
EXERCISE BALL WITH DUMBBELLS
Quadriceps, hamstrings, gluteals

Beginning Position

1. Grasp dumbbells with elbows extended and stand erect with feet about hip-width apart and parallel to each other.
2. Position dumbbells with palms facing outside surfaces of thighs and elbows straight.
3. Place exercise ball between back and wall with feet far enough from wall so that knees are directly over the feet in down position.

Downward Movement Phase

1. Keep head up, eyes fixed straight ahead, shoulders back, torso erect, and weight on entire foot throughout exercise.
2. Squat slowly until thighs are parallel to floor, rolling ball between the back and wall as you descend.
3. Inhale throughout downward movement.

Upward Movement Phase

1. Begin upward movement by slowly straightening knees and hips, rolling ball between the back and wall as you ascend.
2. Exhale throughout upward movement phase.

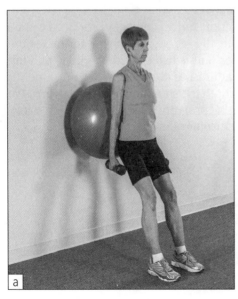
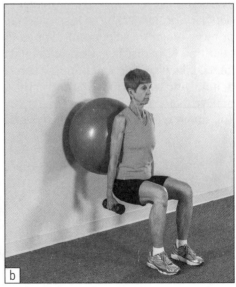

HEEL PULL: EXERCISE BALL
Hamstrings, hip flexors

Beginning Position

1. Lie faceup on floor with legs extended and heels planted firmly on top of an exercise ball.
2. Place the palms of the hands on floor next to hips.

Backward Movement Phase

1. Pull ball toward hips slowly by flexing knees toward chest.
2. Exhale throughout backward movement phase.

Forward Movement Phase

1. Return ball slowly until legs are extended.
2. Inhale throughout forward movement phase.

Note: Do not lift hips off the floor during the heel pull exercise.

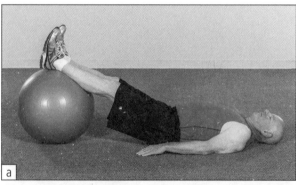

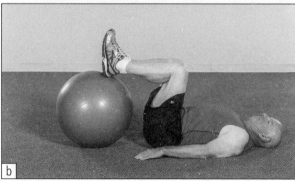

LEG LIFT: EXERCISE BALL
Quadriceps, hip flexors, rectus abdominis

Beginning Position

1. Lie faceup on floor with knees flexed and feet pressed against the sides of exercise ball.
2. Place hands on floor next to hips.

Upward Movement Phase

1. Lift ball upward slowly by extending knees until legs are straight.
2. Exhale throughout lifting movement phase.

Downward Movement Phase

1. Lower ball slowly to floor by flexing knees.
2. Inhale throughout lowering movement phase.

Note: Try to keep thighs in the same position while you lift and lower the exercise ball.

Leg Exercise

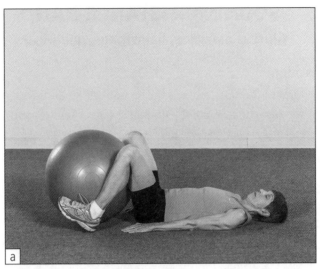

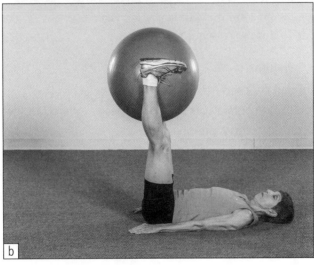

SQUAT: RESISTANCE BAND
Gluteus maximus, hamstrings, quadriceps

Beginning Position

1. Grasp handles of band with palms facing each other and alongside thighs.
2. Stand on top of middle of band with feet shoulder-width apart.
3. Squat so that thighs are at a 45-degree angle to floor.
4. Gather slack of resistance band between feet so that band is taut.
5. Slightly arch your back with shoulders back and chest out so back is flat and torso is erect.

Upward Movement

1. Extend hips and knees at same rate and keep nearly erect flat back position.
2. Keep heels in full contact with floor and knees aligned over feet.
3. Continue upward movement until you are standing.
4. Exhale during this movement phase.

Downward Movement

1. Allow hips and knees to flex at same rate to initial position.
2. Keep heels in full contact with floor and knees aligned over feet.
3. Inhale during this movement phase.

Leg Exercise

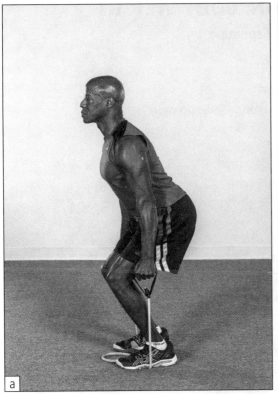 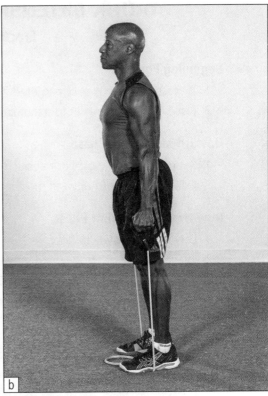

TRUNK EXTENSION: BODY WEIGHT
Erector spinae

Beginning Position
1. Lie facedown on mat or carpeted floor.
2. Place hands under chin to maintain a neutral neck position.

Upward Movement Phase
1. Raise chest slowly off floor about 30 degrees.
2. Exhale throughout upward movement phase.

Downward Movement Phase
1. Lower chest slowly to floor.
2. Inhale throughout downward movement phase.

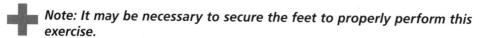 *Note: It may be necessary to secure the feet to properly perform this exercise.*

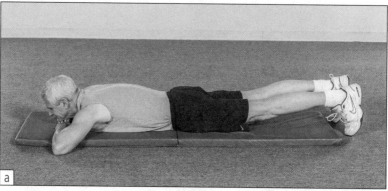

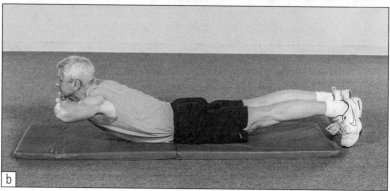

TRUNK EXTENSION: EXERCISE BALL
Erector spinae

Beginning Position

1. Lie facedown on ball with navel positioned on top of ball.
2. Place toes on floor at least 12 inches (30 cm) apart with knees straight (or nearly straight).
3. Clasp hands behind head.

Upward Movement

1. Keeping toes on floor, lift torso until it is straight (or nearly arched) and chest is no longer in contact with top of ball.
2. Exhale during this movement phase.

Downward Movement

1. Allow torso to lower to initial position.
2. Inhale during this movement phase.

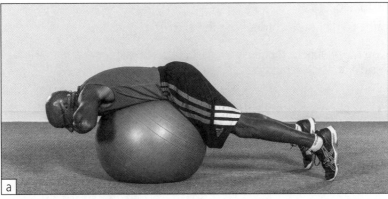

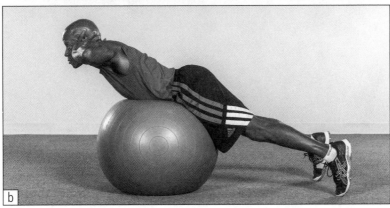

TWISTING TRUNK CURL: BODY WEIGHT

Rectus abdominis, rectus femoris, hip flexors, obliques

Beginning Position

1. Lie faceup on mat or carpeted floor.
2. Place hands behind head to maintain a neutral neck position.

Upward Movement Phase

1. Raise upper back about 30 degrees off floor and keep trunk curled throughout exercise.
2. Lift both legs off floor with right leg straight and left leg bent.
3. Twist torso to left and pull left leg back until right elbow touches left knee.
4. Reverse leg positions and concurrently twist torso to right, pulling right leg back until left elbow touches right knee. Exhale during this movement phase.

Downward Movement Phase

1. Complete as many twisting trunk curls as possible, then lower legs and upper back to floor.
2. Breathe continuously throughout the exercise.

Note: If you are unable to touch elbow to knee, just twist torso and pull knee back as far as possible on each repetition.

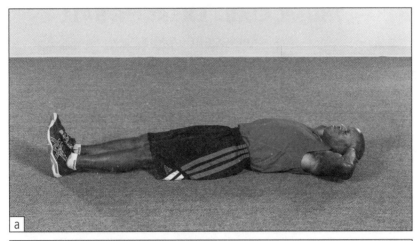

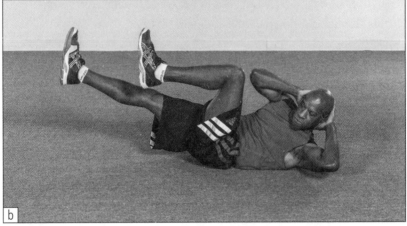

TRUNK CURL: EXERCISE BALL
Rectus abdominis

Beginning Position

1. Lie faceup on ball with feet flat on floor and lower back on ball.
2. Place hands behind head to maintain a neutral neck position.

Upward Movement Phase

1. Raise upper back slowly about 30 degrees off exercise ball.
2. Exhale throughout upward movement phase.

Downward Movement Phase

1. Lower upper back slowly until it is in full contact with exercise ball.
2. Inhale throughout downward movement phase.

Note: This exercise is similar to a standard trunk curl, but the exercise ball increases the movement range and requires more core stabilization from the core muscles.

Core Exercise

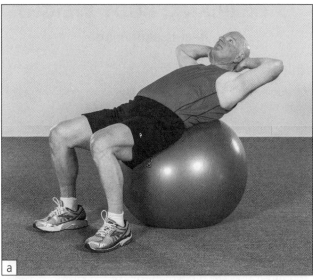

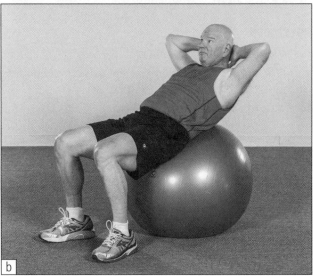

SIDE PLANK: BODY WEIGHT
Rectus abdominis

Beginning Position

1. Lie on right side with only right forearm and right side of hips and legs touching the floor mat.
2. Place left arm along left side of body.
3. Position left leg on top of right leg so they are even with each other.

Upward Movement

1. Contract core muscles to lift hips straight up until whole body is in a straight line suspended off floor.
2. Keep outside of right foot in contact with floor.
3. Do not allow other body segments to sag forward or backward.
4. Exhale throughout upward movement phase.

Downward Movement

1. Allow torso to lower to initial position.
2. Turn over to left side for next set and repeat same movements with outside of left foot in contact with floor during exercise.
3. Inhale during this movement phase.

Core Exercise

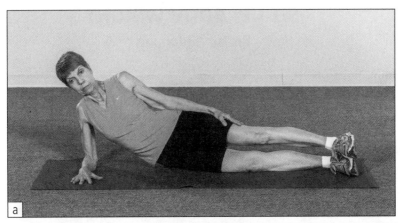

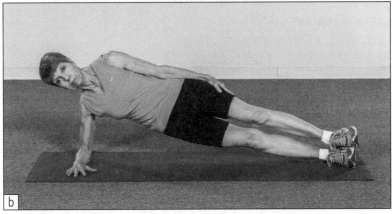

SIT-UP: BODY WEIGHT
Rectus abdominis

Beginning Position
1. Lie faceup on a mat or carpeted floor.
2. Flex knees and cross arms over chest or abdomen.

Upward Movement
1. Curl torso toward thighs until upper back is off the mat.
2. Keep feet flat on mat or floor.
3. Exhale throughout upward movement phase.

Downward Movement
1. Allow torso to uncurl to initial position.
2. Do not let hips lift off mat or floor.
3. Inhale during this movement phase.

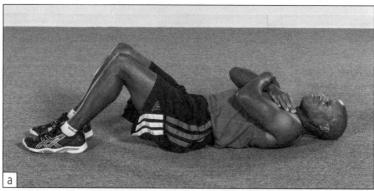

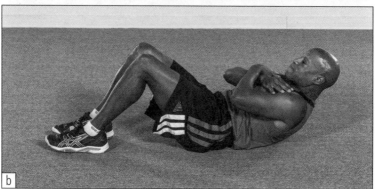

CHEST PRESS: RESISTANCE BAND

Pectoralis major, triceps, anterior deltoids

Beginning Position

1. Grasp handles of band with palms facing forward.
2. Evenly wrap band around torso at midchest level.
3. Stand erect with feet shoulder-width apart and knees slightly flexed.
4. Move handles to sides of torso at midchest height.

Forward Movement Phase

1. Push handles forward from chest until elbows are fully extended.
2. Keep arms parallel to floor and keep the rest of your body stationary.
3. Exhale throughout forward movement phase.

Backward Movement Phase

1. Allow elbows to flex to initial position.
2. Keep arms parallel to floor and keep the rest of your body stationary.
3. Inhale during this movement phase.

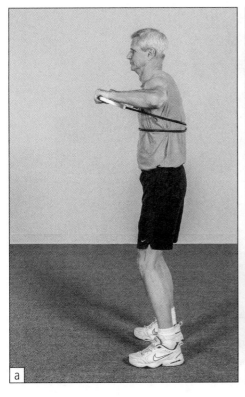 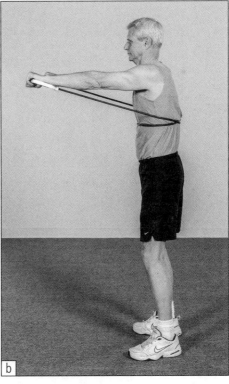

PUSH-UP: EXERCISE BALL
Pectoralis major, anterior deltoids, triceps, rectus abdominis

Beginning Position

1. Assume standard push-up position with hands on floor slightly wider than shoulder-width apart.
2. Place ankles on top of exercise ball with a straight body position.

Downward Movement Phase

1. Lower chest toward floor while maintaining a straight body position.
2. Inhale throughout lowering movement.

Upward Movement Phase

1. Press body upward until arms are fully extended.
2. Exhale throughout the pressing movement.

Note: This exercise is similar to a standard push-up, but use of the exercise ball requires additional core stabilization from the core muscles.

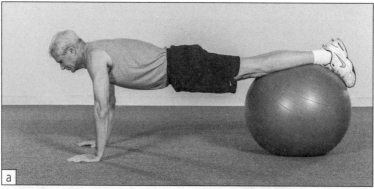

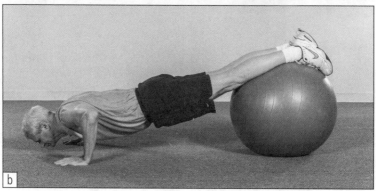

BAR DIP: BODY WEIGHT
Pectoralis major, anterior deltoids, triceps

Beginning Position
1. While facing forward, grasp dip bars with palms facing down, elbows fully extended.
2. Maintain straight body position throughout the exercise.

Downward Movement Phase
1. Lower body slowly until elbows are flexed to 90 degrees.
2. Inhale throughout downward movement phase.

Upward Movement Phase
1. Press body upward until elbows are extended.
2. Exhale throughout upward movement phase.

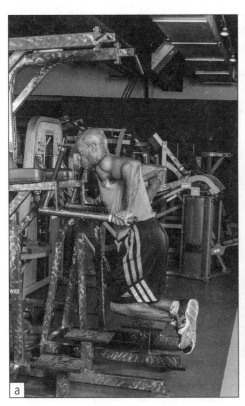 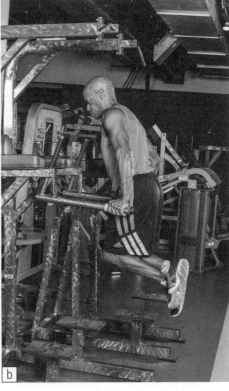

LATERAL RAISE: RESISTANCE BAND
Deltoids

Beginning Position

1. Grasp handles of band with palms facing each other.
2. Stand on top of middle of band with feet shoulder-width apart.
3. Move arms and handles to outside of thighs with palms facing inward.

Upward Movement Phase

1. Lift handles up and out to sides with hands, forearms, elbows, and upper arms rising together. Do not shrug shoulders to help lift the handles.
2. Keep body erect with knees slightly flexed and feet flat on floor.
3. Continue lifting handles until upper arms are parallel to floor or nearly level with shoulders.
4. Exhale during this movement phase.

Downward Movement Phase

1. Allow handles to lower to initial position.
2. Keep body erect with knees slightly flexed and feet flat on floor.
3. Inhale during this movement phase.

Shoulder Exercise

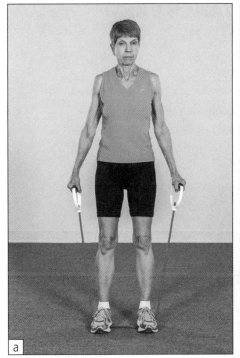

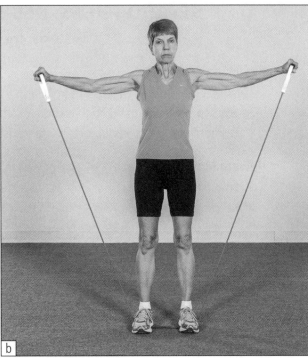

SEATED PRESS: RESISTANCE BAND
Deltoids, triceps

Beginning Position

1. Sit erect on floor with legs out in front.
2. Position body and band so that you are sitting on the middle of band.
3. Position handles to line up with the ears, palms facing forward.

Upward Movement Phase

1. Push handles upward until elbows are fully extended.
2. Keep body erect with wrists straight and directly above shoulders.
3. Exhale during this movement phase.

Downward Movement Phase

1. Allow handles to lower to the initial position.
2. Keep body erect and wrists straight while allowing handles to return to initial position.
3. Inhale during this movement phase.

Shoulder Exercise

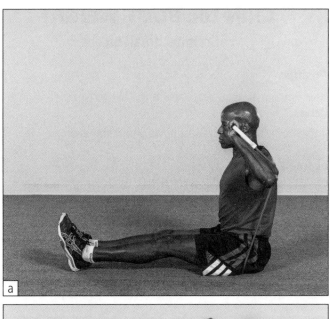

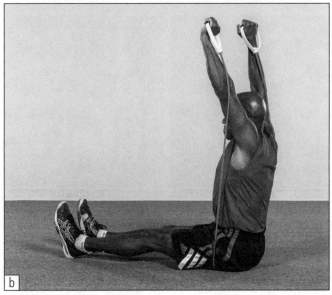

CHIN-UP: BODY WEIGHT
Latissimus dorsi, biceps

Beginning Position

1. Grasp chin-up bar with underhand grip, hands shoulder-width apart, elbows fully extended.
2. Maintain a straight body position throughout the exercise.

Upward Movement Phase

1. Lift body upward until chin is above bar.
2. Exhale throughout upward movement phase.

Downward Movement Phase

1. Lower body slowly until elbows are fully extended.
2. Inhale throughout downward movement phase.

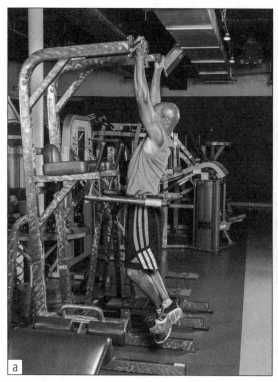
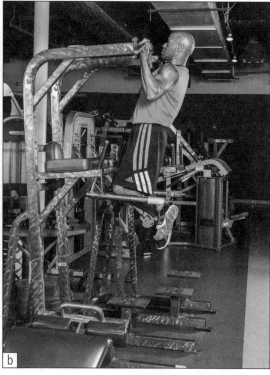

UPRIGHT ROW: RESISTANCE BAND

Deltoids, upper trapezius

Beginning Position

1. Assume a hip-width stance with feet on resistance band and palms close to and facing front of thighs.
2. Stand erect with knees slightly flexed.
3. Maintain a straight body position throughout the exercise.

Upward Movement Phase

1. Pull handles along abdomen and chest toward your chin.
2. Keep elbows pointed out to the sides as the handles move along torso.
3. Do not lift up heels or swing handles to move outward or up.
4. At the highest position, elbows should be level with or slightly higher than shoulders and wrists.
5. Exhale throughout the upward movement.

Downward Movement Phase

1. Lower handles to the initial position.
2. Keep torso and knees in the same position; do not lean forward during lowering phase.
3. Inhale during lowering phase.

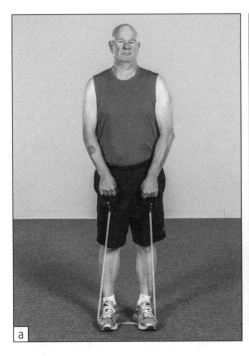
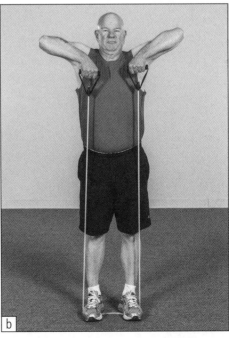

SEATED ROW: RESISTANCE BAND
Latissimus dorsi, biceps

Beginning Position

1. Wrap resistance band securely around the soles of feet, and grasp it with palms facing each other and elbows fully extended.
2. Assume an erect position (torso perpendicular to the floor) with knees slightly flexed.
3. The resistance band should be nearly taut; use one of a shorter length or widen the stance.

Backward Movement Phase

1. Flex elbows and pull handles toward chest while maintaining an erect position.
2. Exhale during this movement phase.

Forward Movement Phase

1. Allow the elbows to fully extend back to the starting position while maintaining an erect torso position.
2. Inhale during this movement phase.

Upper-Back Exercise

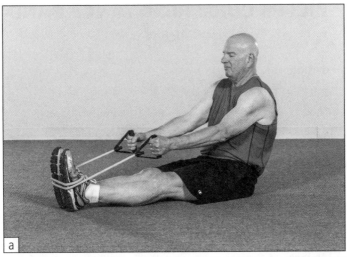

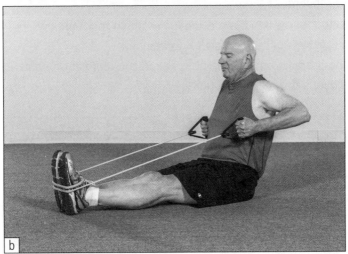

BICEPS CURL: RESISTANCE BAND
Biceps

Beginning Position

1. Grasp handles of resistance band with palms facing forward.
2. Stand on top of middle of band with feet shoulder-width apart.
3. Move arms and handles to outside of thighs.

Upward Movement Phase

1. Flex elbows to raise the handles toward shoulders.
2. Keep body erect with knees slightly flexed and feet flat on floor.
3. Exhale during this movement phase.

Downward Movement

1. Allow elbows to extend to move handles down to initial position.
2. Lower handles until elbows are fully extended.
3. Keep body erect with knees slightly flexed and feet flat on floor.
4. Inhale during this movement phase.

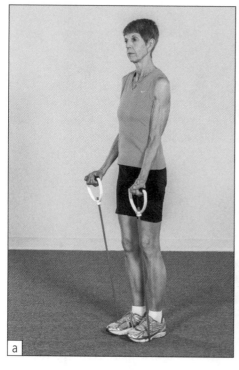
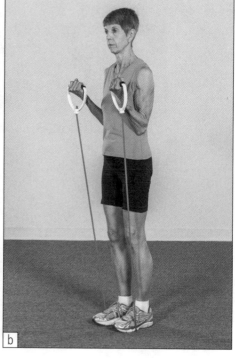

BENCH DIP: EXERCISE BALL
Triceps, pectoralis major, anterior deltoids

Beginning Position

1. Place heels of hands on bench with elbows extended and heels of feet on exercise ball with legs extended so that hips are in front of bench.
2. Maintain an L body position throughout the exercise.

Downward Movement Phase

1. Lower hips slowly toward floor until elbows are flexed to 90 degrees.
2. Inhale throughout downward movement phase.

Upward Movement Phase

1. Press body upward slowly until elbows are fully extended.
2. Exhale throughout upward movement phase.

Note: This exercise is similar to standard bench dips, but using the exercise ball requires additional core stabilization from the midsection.

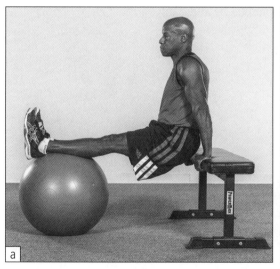
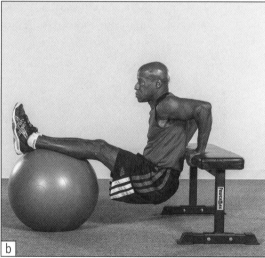

ONE-ARM TRICEPS EXTENSION: RESISTANCE BAND
Triceps

Beginning Position
1. Grasp handles of band with palms facing upward.
2. Sit erect on a floor mat with legs out in front.
3. Position body and band so that you are sitting on top of the middle of the band.
4. Flex elbows to move your arms and handles behind head and upper back with palms facing forward.

Upward Movement Phase
1. Extend left elbow until hand is over your head.
2. Do not let wrist flex, and keep upper arm next to your head.
3. Exhale during this movement phase.

Downward Movement Phase
1. Allow left elbow to flex to move the handle down to the initial position.
2. Repeat exercise with right arm and continue by alternating arms.
3. Inhale during this movement phase.

Arm Exercise

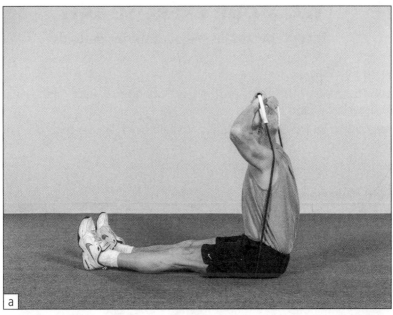

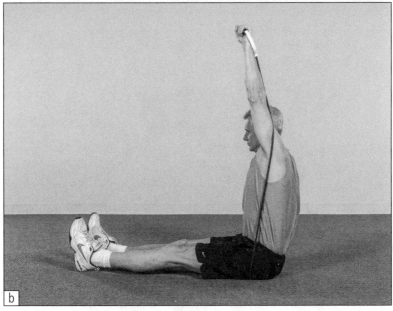

WALK-OUT: EXERCISE BALL

Triceps, pectoralis major, anterior deltoids

Beginning Position

1. Assume standard push-up position with hands on floor slightly wider than shoulder-width apart.
2. Place ankles on top of exercise ball and maintain a straight body position parallel to floor.
3. Maintain straight body position throughout exercise.

Backward Movement Phase

1. Walk hands backward toward exercise ball, allowing legs to roll backward over ball.
2. Breathe continuously throughout backward movement phase.

Forward Movement Phase

1. Walk hands forward away from exercise ball, allowing legs to roll forward over ball.
2. Breathe continuously throughout forward movement.

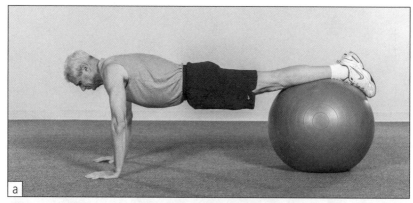

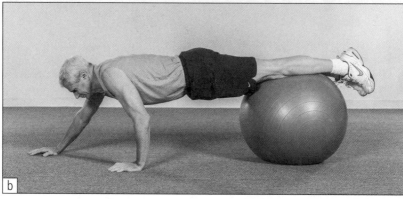

SHRUG: RESISTANCE BAND

Upper trapezius

Beginning Position

1. Establish a hip-width stance with feet standing on resistance band.
2. Grasp handles with palms facing thighs, arms at sides and fully extended.
3. Stand erect and keep arms straight throughout exercise.

Upward Movement Phase

1. Elevate (shrug) shoulders as high as possible toward ears in unison.
2. Exhale throughout shrugging movement phase.

Downward Movement Phase

1. Allow handles to slowly lower to starting position in unison.
2. Inhale throughout lowering movement phase.

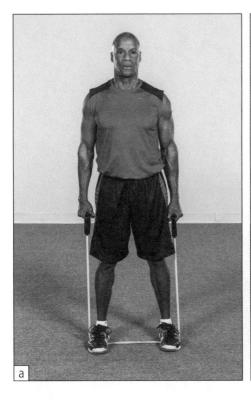
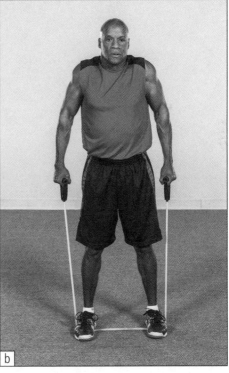

9

Basic Training Programs

This chapter presents several sample resistance training programs for beginning exercisers and for those who prefer a basic strength training protocol. There are programs for people who prefer to use resistance machines (exercises described in chapter 6); those who prefer to work with free weights (exercises described in chapter 7); and those who prefer to train with body weight, exercise balls, and resistance bands (exercises described in chapter 8). Two training programs are presented for each mode of resistance exercise: a brief workout (6 exercises) and a standard training routine (12 exercises). Begin with the training program that best accommodates your preference for resistance equipment and time availability, and feel free to substitute other exercises if you are unable to perform any of those presented in the tables. For example, you may select other exercises performed with the same type of resistance equipment (e.g., free weights), or you may perform the same exercise with a different type of resistance equipment (e.g., resistance bands).

Regardless of which basic training program you select, start with a training load that is 60 to 70 percent of the heaviest weight that you can lift for one repetition (1RM) with proper technique. Because a fairly predictable relationship exists between the resistance you use and the number of repetitions you are able to perform, it is not necessary to determine your maximum load for each exercise. As you may recall from chapter 3, most people are capable of completing about 12 repetitions with 70 percent of maximum load and about 16 repetitions with 60 percent of maximum load in most exercises. With this in mind, experiment with each exercise in the program you select to determine the load that will result in 12 to 15 repetitions when giving a good effort. The load determined will serve as your training load. Continue training with this load until you can complete 16 repetitions. When you can perform 16 repetitions with proper technique during two consecutive workouts, you are ready to progress to a heavier training load (an increase of about 5 percent).

The basic fitness training program is predicated on performing one good set of each exercise with an appropriate resistance. If time is not a limiting factor, you may perform a warm-up set of each exercise using 50 to 60 percent of the training load. As you progress, you may want to add a second set of some or all of the training exercises presented in the program. Just be sure that the training loads enable you to complete 12 to 16 repetitions of each exercise set. We recommend using the same resistance for both exercise sets.

The basic fitness training program features one or two sets of each exercise (plus a warm-up set if desired) to strengthen the major muscle groups. A rest period of

60 to 90 seconds should be sufficient for recovering from the previous exercise set and for reducing the cumulative effects of muscle fatigue as you perform your workout. You should train reasonably hard, but the final repetition in your exercise set should not be at a do-or-die level of difficulty. Simply train to the point of momentary muscle fatigue, which means you would be hard pressed to complete another repetition with proper technique if you tried to do so.

EXERCISE SELECTION

When we select resistance exercises for basic strength training programs, first we feature one multiple-muscle pushing exercise that concurrently works the major pushing muscles in the upper body (pectoralis major, anterior deltoids, triceps). We realize that muscles can only pull, but the result of these coordinated muscle contractions is a pushing action (movement away from the body). The best-upper body pushing exercises are machine chest press, barbell bench press, dumbbell bench press, resistance band chest press, and body-weight push-up. You will find one or more of these upper-body pushing exercises in all of our recommended basic strength training programs in this chapter.

Second, we feature one multiple-muscle pulling exercise that simultaneously works the major pulling muscles in the upper body (latissimus dorsi, posterior deltoids, biceps, middle trapezius, rhomboids). Again, all muscles pull, but the result of these coordinated muscle contractions is a pulling action (movement toward the body). The best upper-body pulling exercises are machine seated row, machine pulldown, dumbbell one-arm row, resistance band seated row, and body-weight chin-up. You will find one or more of these upper-body pulling exercises in all of our recommended basic strength training programs in this chapter.

Third, we feature one multiple-muscle pushing exercise that simultaneously works the major muscles in the hips and thighs (gluteals, quadriceps, hamstrings). Because of the unique biomechanics of the hip and thigh musculature, the quadriceps muscles produce extension at the knee joints, while the opposing hamstring and gluteal muscles produce extension at the hip joints. That is, these seemingly antagonistic muscle groups actually work together to achieve coordinated pushing actions of the legs. The most effective exercises for simultaneously working these large muscle groups are machine leg press, barbell squat, dumbbell squat, and resistance band squat. You will find one of these leg pushing exercises in all of our recommended basic strength training programs in this chapter.

Although all of the recommended multiple-muscle exercises for upper-body pushing movements, upper-body pulling movements, and leg pushing movements require some degree of trunk stabilization, the next phase of exercise selection focuses on the core muscles (rectus abdominis, erector spinae, external and internal obliques). The rectus abdominis muscles, typically referred to as the abs, are responsible for trunk flexion and are best addressed by machine abdominal flexion and body-weight trunk curl. Conversely, the erector spinae muscles of the lower back are responsible for trunk extension. The best exercises for safely strengthening these muscles are machine low back extension and body-weight trunk extension. The external and internal oblique muscles work together to produce clockwise trunk rotation (right internal obliques and left external obliques) and counterclockwise trunk rotation (left internal obliques and right external obliques). The best exercises for safely strengthening these four integrated muscles are the machine rotary torso and the body-weight twisting trunk curl. You will find these exercises for the core muscles in our recommended basic strength training programs in this chapter.

Once you have addressed the major muscle groups of the upper body, legs, and trunk, you will add exercises for other muscle groups that have not received as much (or any) stimulus from the primary exercises. For example, although the shoulder muscles are involved in pushing exercises, such as bench press, they are better targeted with overhead movements such as machine shoulder press, barbell incline press, dumbbell press, and resistance band press.

Likewise, although the recommended pushing exercises use the triceps, these muscles can be better isolated with the machine triceps extension and dumbbell lying triceps extension exercises. In a similar manner, the recommended pulling exercises use the biceps, but these muscles can be better isolated with the machine biceps curl, dumbbell incline curl, and resistance band curl.

When possible, you should include exercises for the other major muscle groups of the thighs. These are the hip adductor muscles of the inner thigh and the hip abductor muscles of the outer thigh. The best exercises for working these muscles through their full range of motion are machine hip adduction and machine hip abduction exercises. We have included these exercises in our standard machine strength training machine routine (see program 9.2). Unfortunately, it is difficult to isolate these muscles with free weights and challenging to work these muscles with bands, so we have not included hip adduction and hip abduction exercises for these training modalities.

We hope that you will find each of the basic training programs effective for strengthening your major muscle groups. Of course, you will attain a more comprehensive workout if you are able to do one of the standard routines because these training programs have twice as many exercises as the brief workouts (12 exercises versus 6 exercises).

PROTOCOLS FOR BASIC STRENGTH TRAINING

As previously mentioned, this chapter covers two types of workouts: brief and standard. The brief workout program, designed for each type of training equipment, features six exercises that address most of the major muscle groups and requires less training time than the standard programs. These programs may be more appropriate for beginning participants and time-pressured exercisers. If you are just starting to strength train and your average score in chapter 2 was 5.0, 5.3, or 5.6 on the strength assessments, we suggest that you begin with one of the shorter (brief workout) exercise programs and progress to a more comprehensive training program once you feel confident. The standard workout programs in this chapter are 12 exercises that are more appropriately undertaken by those with some training experience but whose average score in chapter 2 was 5.0, 5.3, or 5.6. The standard workout programs provide you with a comprehensive exercise experience but require longer training sessions. The following sections present both brief workouts and standard training routines using resistance machines, free weights, or combined body weight, exercise ball, and resistance bands.

PROGRAM 9.1: BRIEF WORKOUT

Program 9.1 is an abbreviated machine workout that uses six standard exercises that collectively work most of the major muscle groups. The first four exercises are linear movements that cumulatively address most of the muscles of the leg, upper body, and upper arm. The last two (rotary movement) exercises target the abdominal and low back muscles that are critical to core strength.

The six basic exercises in the short strength training program actually provide a pretty comprehensive workout, including the front thighs, rear thighs, hips, chest, upper back, shoulders, front arms, rear arms, neck and midsection (core).

If you perform one set of each exercise, you should complete this workout in approximately 12 to 15 minutes; it will take approximately twice as long (24 to 30 minutes) if you perform a preliminary warm-up set or do two sets of each exercise. Perform the exercises in the recommended order, which involves training the larger muscle groups first, then the smaller ones. This arrangement of exercises alternates pushing with pulling movements for best results. The table presents the program 9.1 exercises along with general guidelines for training loads (resistance), repetitions, sets, repetition speed, and recovery time.

Machine Training

Program 9.1—Machine Training (Brief Workout)

Exercise	Muscle group	Page #
1. Leg press	Quadriceps, hamstrings, gluteals	62
2. Chest press	Pectoralis major, anterior deltoids, triceps	71
3. Seated row	Latissimus dorsi, posterior deltoids, biceps, middle trapezius, rhomboids, teres major	79
4. Shoulder press	Deltoids, triceps, upper trapezius	74
5. Abdominal flexion	Core: Rectus abdominis	68
6. Low back extension	Core: Erector spinae	67

Training load	Repetitions	Sets	Repetition speed	Recovery time
60-70% max	12-16	1-2	4-6 sec	60-90 sec

PROGRAM 9.2: STANDARD ROUTINE

Program 9.2 is a machine workout that includes 12 excellent resistance exercises that collectively work the most important major muscle groups. The three leg exercises involve the key muscles of the hips and thighs. The six upper-body exercises address the prominent muscles in the chest, upper back, shoulders, and arms. The three core exercises target the lower back and midsection. Five of these exercises are linear actions (straight movements) that work at least two major muscle groups simultaneously. The other seven exercises are rotary actions (curved movements) that focus on specific muscle groups.

Note that most of the strength training exercises in this program are sequenced to alternately address opposing muscle groups. For example, the chest press (an upper-body pushing exercise) is followed by the seated row (an upper-body pulling exercise). Similarly, the shoulder press (another upper-body pushing exercise) is followed by the lat pulldown (another upper-body pulling exercise). Likewise, the triceps extension exercise for the rear arm muscles is followed by the biceps curl exercise for the muscles at the front of the arm, and the abdominal flexion exercise for the front core muscles is followed by the low back extension exercise for the rear core muscles. By training in this exercise pattern, you will attain overall and balanced muscular conditioning in a relatively efficient manner.

Program 9.2 should take only 24 to 30 minutes if you perform one set of each exercise. If you perform a preliminary warm-up set or add a second set the workout will last approximately 48 to 60 minutes. Perform the exercises in the order listed, progressing from larger to smaller muscle groups. The table presents the recommended exercises for program 9.2 as well as general guidelines for the training loads to use, repetitions to complete, sets to perform, and repetition speed and recovery periods.

Machine Training

Program 9.2—Machine Training (Standard Routine)

Exercise	Muscle group	Page #
1. Leg press	Quadriceps, hamstrings, gluteals	62
2. Hip adduction	Hip adductors	64
3. Hip abduction	Hip abductors	65
4. Chest press	Pectoralis major, anterior deltoids, triceps	71
5. Seated row	Latissimus dorsi, posterior deltoids, biceps, middle trapezius, rhomboids, teres major	79
6. Shoulder press	Deltoids, triceps, upper trapezius	74
7. Lat pulldown	Latissimus dorsi, biceps, teres major	78
8. Triceps extension	Triceps	85
9. Biceps curl	Biceps	84
10. Abdominal flexion	Core: Rectus abdominis	68
11. Low back extension	Core: Erector spinae	67
12. Rotary torso	Core: External obliques, internal obliques, rectus abdominis	69

Training Load	Repetitions	Sets	Repetition speed	Recovery time
60-70% max	12-16	1-2	4-6 sec	60-90 sec

PROGRAM 9.3: BRIEF WORKOUT

Program 9.3 is an abbreviated workout that uses four basic free-weight exercises and two body-weight exercises to train the most important major muscle groups. The four free-weight exercises are linear actions (straight movements) that address the most important muscles of the legs, chest, upper back, shoulders, and arms. The two body-weight exercises are rotary actions that target the major muscles of the core. As in our other sample training programs, you will alternate pushing and pulling exercises to enhance the efficiency of your workouts.

You should be able to complete the brief workout in 12 to 15 minutes if you perform one set of each exercise. The workout should take about twice as long (24 to 30 minutes) if you perform a preliminary warm-up set or add a second set of each exercise. If you prefer dumbbell training, you may substitute dumbbells for the squat, bench press, and seated press exercises. You may also use kettlebells in the squat and one-arm row. Follow the recommended exercise sequence as closely as possible. The table presents the program 9.3 exercises and general training guidelines for resistance, repetitions, sets, repetition speed, and recovery time.

Program 9.3—Free-Weight Training (Brief Workout)

Exercise	Muscle group	Page #
1. Barbell or dumbbell squat*	Quadriceps, hamstrings, gluteals	94, 92
2. Barbell or dumbbell bench press	Pectoralis major, anterior deltoids, triceps	112, 110
3. Dumbbell one-arm row*	Latissimus dorsi, posterior deltoids, biceps, middle trapezius, rhomboids, teres major	126
4. Barbell standing press or dumbbell seated press	Deltoids, triceps, upper trapezius	122, 119
5. Body-weight twisting trunk curl**	Core: rectus abdominis, external obliques, internal obliques, hip flexors, rectus femoris	152
6. Body-weight trunk extension**	Core: erector spinae	150

Training load	Repetitions	Sets	Repetition speed	Recovery time
60-70% max	12-16	1-2	4-6 sec	60-90 sec

*May also be performed using kettlebells.

**Body-weight exercises: As many repetitions as necessary to fatigue the target muscles.

PROGRAM 9.4: STANDARD ROUTINE

Program 9.4 is a free-weight workout that features 12 basic exercises that collectively train most of the major muscle groups; it is similar to the machine training exercises in program 9.2. The leg exercise involves the main muscles of the hips and thighs. The nine upper-body exercises address the prominent muscles in the chest, upper back, shoulders, and arms. The two body-weight core exercises target the abdominal and low back muscles. This exercise program involves linear actions (straight movements) that work at least two major muscle groups simultaneously and rotary actions (curved movements) that focus on specific muscle groups.

Note that the upper-body exercises are sequenced to alternately address opposing muscle groups. For example, the barbell bench press (an upper-body pushing exercise) is followed by the dumbbell one-arm row (an upper-body pulling exercise). The barbell incline press (another upper-body pushing exercise) is followed by the dumbbell pullover (another upper-body pulling exercise). Next, the dumbbell fly for the chest muscles is followed by the dumbbell reverse fly for the upper-back muscles. The dumbbell incline curl for the front of the arms is followed by the dumbbell lying triceps extension for the back of the arms. Likewise, the body-weight twisting trunk curl for the abdominal muscles is followed by the body-weight trunk extension for the low back muscles. By training in this exercise pattern, you attain overall muscular conditioning in a more efficient manner.

Program 9.4 should take about 24 to 30 minutes if you perform one set of each exercise. If you perform a preliminary warm-up set or add a second exercise set, the workout will take approximately 48 to 60 minutes. If you prefer dumbbell training, you may substitute dumbbells for the squat, bench press, and incline press exercises. You may also use kettlebells for the squat, one-arm row, shrug, and heel raise. You should have best results by performing the exercises in the recommended sequence. The program 9.4 exercises and general training guidelines for resistance, repetitions, sets, repetition speed, and recovery time are presented in the following table. Be sure to incorporate a spotter when performing the barbell squat, barbell bench press, and barbell incline press.

Program 9.4—Free-Weight Training (Standard Routine)

Exercise	Muscle group	Page #
1. Barbell or dumbbell squat*	Quadriceps, hamstrings, gluteals	94, 102
2. Barbell or dumbbell bench press	Pectoralis major, anterior deltoids, triceps	112, 110
3. Dumbbell one-arm row*	Latissimus dorsi, posterior deltoids, biceps, middle trapezius, rhomboids, teres major	126
4. Barbell or dumbbell incline press	Pectoralis major, anterior deltoids, triceps	114, 116
5. Dumbbell pullover	Latissimus dorsi, teres major, triceps	124
6. Dumbbell chest fly	Pectoralis major, anterior deltoids, serratus anterior	109
7. Dumbbell reverse fly	Latissimus dorsi, middle trapezius, rhomboids, triceps	129
8. Dumbbell seated press	Deltoids, triceps, upper trapezius	119
9. Dumbbell incline curl	Biceps	132
10. Dumbbell lying triceps extension	Triceps	136
11. Body-weight twisting trunk curl**	Core: rectus abdominis, external obliques, internal obliques, hip flexors, rectus femoris	152
12. Body-weight trunk extension**	Core: erector spinae	150

Training load	Repetitions	Sets	Repetition speed	Recovery time
60-70% max	12-16	1-2	4-6 sec	60-90 sec

*May also be performed using kettlebells.

**Body-weight exercises: As many repetitions as necessary to fatigue the target muscles.

PROGRAM 9.5: BRIEF WORKOUT

Program 9.5 is an efficient training session using various forms of exercise and resistance. To enhance training intensity in the body-weight exercises, performed with or without an exercise ball, simply increase the number of repetitions of each exercise set. The resistance band exercises use a non-gravity-based resistance that increases as the elastic band or rubber tubing is stretched (see discussion in chapter 4). Unlike machine weight stacks, free weights, and body-weight resistance that are lifted upward against the force of gravity, elastic bands provide a gradually increasing resistance in any direction that they are extended. Elastic bands and rubber tubing are available in various thicknesses so that you can progressively increase the exercise resistance by changing to thicker bands or tubes. You should select an appropriately sized resistance band or rubber tube to permit one or two sets of 12 to 16 repetitions for each training exercise. When you can complete 16 repetitions with correct technique, you should progress to a thicker band or tube that provides slightly more resistance.

The six exercises in the brief workout include three with body weight (push-up, twisting trunk curl, trunk extension) and three with resistance bands (squat, seated row, shoulder press). These six basic exercises involve most of the major muscle groups: First, the resistance band squat works the quadriceps, hamstrings, and gluteal muscles. The body-weight push-up using an exercise ball addresses the pectoralis major, anterior deltoid, and triceps muscles as well as the front core musculature. The next exercise, resistance band seated row, involves the opposing muscle groups of the upper back, rear shoulders, and biceps as well as the rear core musculature. The fourth exercise, resistance band shoulder press, works the shoulder, triceps, and upper trapezius muscles. The final two exercises address the core musculature: The body-weight twisting trunk curl targets the rectus abdominis and oblique muscles, and the body-weight trunk extension targets the erector spinae muscles.

Program 9.5 should require about 12 to 15 minutes if you perform one set of each exercise. Completing two sets of each exercise will extend your training session to approximately 24 to 30 minutes. It is advisable to perform the exercises in the recommended order of larger to smaller muscle groups, alternating pushing and pulling movements for best results. The table presents the program 9.5 exercises along with general guidelines for resistance, repetitions, sets, repetition speed, and recovery time.

Body-Weight, Exercise Ball, and Resistance Band Training

Program 9.5—Body-Weight, Exercise Ball, and Resistance Band Training (Brief Workout)

Exercise	Muscle group	Page #
1. Resistance band squat	Quadriceps, hamstrings, gluteals	148
2. Body-weight push-up: exercise ball*	Pectoralis major, anterior deltoids, triceps, rectus abdominis	160
3. Resistance band seated row	Latissimus dorsi, posterior deltoids, biceps, middle trapezius, rhomboids, erector spinae	168
4. Resistance band seated press	Deltoids, triceps, upper trapezius	164
5. Body-weight twisting trunk curl*	Core: rectus abdominis, external obliques, internal obliques, hip flexors, rectus femoris	152
6. Body-weight trunk extension: exercise ball*	Core: erector spinae	151

Training load	Repetitions	Sets	Repetition speed	Recovery time
60-70% max	12-16	1-2	4-6 sec	60-90 sec

*Body-weight exercises: As many repetitions as necessary to fatigue the target muscles.

PROGRAM 9.6: STANDARD ROUTINE

Program 9.6 provides a basic training protocol of 12 exercises that are performed with body weight, exercise balls, and resistance bands. You should perform body-weight exercises, with or without the use of an exercise ball, for as many repetitions as necessary to fatigue the target muscles. This will most likely require more repetitions in some body-weight exercises, such as trunk curls, than in other body-weight exercises, such as chin-ups. Unlike body-weight exercises, elastic bands and rubber tubes provide external resistance that increases gradually as the material is stretched. Unlike gravity-based free weights, elastic bands and rubber tubes provide resistance in any direction that they are extended, thereby offering greater versatility in exercises. Elastic bands and rubber tubes are available in various thicknesses that enable you to progressively increase the exercise resistance by changing to thicker bands or tubes (see discussion in chapter 4). Ideally, you should train with a band or tube that permits you to perform one or two sets of 12 to 16 repetitions for each exercise. When you can complete 16 repetitions with correct technique, you should progress to a thicker band or tube that provides slightly more resistance.

The 12 recommended exercises feature 4 with resistance bands and 8 with body-weight resistance (including 5 exercises that use an exercise ball). The first exercise is the resistance band squat that works the front and rear thighs. The next two exercises involve both body weight and an exercise ball for the rear thigh and front thigh, respectively. The following three exercises use body-weight resistance to address the upper-body pushing muscles (bench dip and push-up) and the upper-body pulling muscles (chin-up). The next three exercises use resistance bands to further stimulate the upper-body pulling muscles (seated row and curl) and the upper-body pushing muscles (shoulder press). The final three exercises use body-weight resistance to train the front, side, and rear core musculature (trunk curl, trunk extension, and twisting trunk curl).

Program 9.6 training sessions should take about 24 to 30 minutes if you perform one set of each exercise and twice as long (48 to 60 minutes) if you complete two sets of each exercise. It is advisable to perform the exercises in the recommended order of larger to smaller muscle groups, alternating pushing and pulling movements for best results. The table presents the program 9.6 exercises along with general guidelines for resistance, repetitions, sets, repetition speed, and recovery time.

Program 9.6—Body-Weight, Exercise Ball, and Resistance Band Training (Standard Routine)

Exercise	Muscle group	Page #
1. Resistance band squat	Quadriceps, hamstrings, gluteals	148
2. Heel pull: exercise ball	Hamstrings, hip flexors	145
3. Leg lift: exercise ball	Quadriceps, hip flexors, rectus abdominis	146
4. Body-weight bench dip*	Pectoralis major, anterior deltoids, triceps, latissimus dorsi, teres major	171
5. Body-weight chin-up*	Latissimus dorsi, biceps, posterior deltoids, teres major	161
6. Body-weight push-up: exercise ball*	Pectoralis major, anterior deltoids, triceps, rectus abdominis	160
7. Resistance band seated row	Latissimus dorsi, posterior deltoids, biceps, middle trapezius, rhomboids, teres major	168
8. Resistance band seated press	Deltoids, triceps, upper trapezius	164
9. Resistance band biceps curl	Biceps	170
10. Body-weight trunk curl: exercise ball*	Core: rectus abdominis	154
11. Body-weight trunk extension: exercise ball*	Core: erector spinae	151
12. Body-weight twisting trunk curl*	Core: rectus abdominis, external obliques, internal obliques, hip flexors, rectus femoris	152

Training load	Repetitions	Sets	Repetition speed	Recovery time
60-70% max	12-16	1-2	4-6 sec	60-90 sec

*Body-weight exercises: As many repetitions as necessary to fatigue the target muscles.

PROGRESSION OF TRAINING PROGRAM

Whichever training program you select should work well for several weeks or months as you gradually increase the training loads (resistance) and the number of sets to accommodate your increased strength. However, at some point, you will undoubtedly encounter a strength plateau. We define a strength plateau as three consecutive weeks of training during which there is no increase in the number of repetitions performed. For example, if you have completed 14 chest presses with 75 pounds for the past three weeks but have not been capable of performing a 15th repetition, you most likely are in a strength plateau. Upon reaching a strength plateau, you need to change some aspect of your training program rather than do more of the same routine that led to the plateau. You might be able to remediate a strength plateau by taking a week off from training (if you have been working very hard) or simply changing related lifestyle behaviors such as eating and sleeping. In other cases, you may need to replace your present basic training program with one of the more advanced exercise protocols in chapter 10 to stimulate greater muscle response and further strength gains. Although the strength training programs in chapter 10 are more challenging, these advanced workouts should be more effective for attaining higher levels of muscle development.

10

Advanced Training Programs

Either your chapter 2 average strength fitness score was 6.0, 6.3, 6.6, or 7.0, which has directed you to this chapter for advanced training programs, or you have progressed to this training category by completing one of the basic fitness programs in chapter 9. Whichever the case, you should adhere to the advanced training protocols described in this chapter. You will find two advanced exercise programs for training with machines, two programs for using free-weight equipment, and two programs involving body weight, exercise ball, or resistance bands.

Regardless of which advanced training program you select, use a training load of 70 to 80 percent of the weight (or load) you can lift for one repetition. Because a fairly predictable relationship exists between the resistance you use and the number of repetitions you are able to perform, it is not necessary to determine your maximum load for each exercise. As you may recall from chapter 3, most people are capable of completing about 8 repetitions with 80 percent of maximum load and about 12 repetitions with 70 percent of maximum load in most exercises. With this in mind, experiment with each exercise to determine the load that will result in 8 to 11 repetitions when giving a good effort. The resistance determined will serve as your temporary training load. Continue training with this load until you can complete 12 repetitions. When you can perform 12 repetitions with proper technique during two consecutive workouts, you are ready to progress to a heavier training load (about 5 percent more resistance). Training in this double-progressive manner reduces the risk of doing too much too soon and provides regular positive reinforcement for your exercise efforts.

Advanced programs 10.1, 10.3, and 10.5 are high-load and high-volume training protocols of two or three exercise sets using progressively higher resistance. Advanced programs 10.2, 10.4, and 10.6 offer alternative exercise protocols known as high-intensity training. These training techniques require very short recovery periods between successive exercises for the target muscle groups or between extended exercise sets. You should find that one good set of each exercise in programs 10.2, 10.4, and 10.6 is effective for stimulating muscle development.

If you have time, you may perform a warm-up set of each exercise in the advanced training program. Your warm-up set should equal 50 to 60 percent of your training weight load. If you perform multiple-set training in advanced training program 10.1, 10.3, or 10.5, we recommend 90 to 120 seconds of rest between successive sets of the same exercise because this is the approximate time required to replace muscle energy stores after a hard bout of strength training. However, if you perform the high-intensity training techniques in program 10.2, 10.4, or 10.6, we recommend very brief recovery periods (5 to 15 seconds; see bottom of program tables for details) to maximize the effectiveness of the exercises. Although it is not necessary to train to the point of muscle failure (inability of the muscle to continue contraction), you should not terminate your exercise sets before reaching momentary muscle fatigue. Generally, you should continue exercising until you are certain that you cannot complete another repetition with correct technique. If your muscles fatigue in the middle of a repetition, simply stop. Do not compromise correct lifting technique and risk injury in an effort to complete an additional repetition after you have momentary muscle fatigue.

PREVENTING STRENGTH PLATEAUS

Beginning strength trainers make progress at a relatively rapid rate during the first several weeks of resistance exercise. Much of the early-phase gain in strength is due to motor learning, which is essentially neuromuscular facilitation that enhances muscle fiber recruitment and increases muscle force production. Although we have seen consistent increases in muscle strength and size over the first six to nine months of our strength training programs, progress eventually slows and becomes a temporary strength plateau. That is, the basic training protocol no longer produces desirable gains in strength. Rather than be discouraged, take this as a sign that some aspect of your exercise program needs to be changed to stimulate further development of strength. Although this may include a variety of exercise factors, the successful transition from beginning to advanced strength training generally requires a more challenging workout program.

One means for enhancing the muscle-building stimulus is to increase the training volume, which is typically accomplished by performing additional exercise sets. You will note that programs 10.1, 10.3, and 10.5 incorporate multiple sets of each training exercise.

A second means for enhancing the muscle-building stimulus is to increase the training resistance, which is typically achieved by using higher loads and performing fewer repetitions. You will see that programs 10.1, 10.3, and 10.5 involve three sets of each exercise with increasing loads (70%-80%-90% of maximum) and decreasing repetitions (12-8-4 repetitions).

A third procedure for making the workout more productive is to increase the training intensity, or the muscular effort, required for completing each exercise set. Programs 10.2, 10.4, and 10.6 use high-intensity training techniques to stimulate more muscle development.

HIGH-INTENSITY STRENGTH TRAINING

The most common means for performing high-intensity strength training is extending the exercise set with a few postfatigue repetitions. For example, if you complete 10 biceps curls to fatigue with 60 pounds, at the end of this set you have reduced the strength of your biceps muscles to slightly less than 60 pounds. Although you cannot perform another repetition with 60 pounds, you have not totally exhausted your biceps muscles. If you immediately reduce the resistance to 50 pounds, you should be able to perform two to four additional repetitions. We call these post-fatigue repetitions because you have already reached an effective level of biceps muscle fatigue during your first set of curls with 60 pounds. When you complete an immediate extended set of two to four curls with 50 pounds, your biceps muscles experience a deeper level of fatigue and thereby a greater stimulus for muscle development.

We refer to this high-intensity exercise technique as breakdown training because you break down the resistance to essentially match the reduced strength level in the prefatigued muscles. In addition to enhancing the training effect, performing two to four postfatigue repetitions is an efficient exercise technique, requiring only 10 to 20 more seconds to complete the extended set.

A similar procedure for increasing the exercise intensity is known as prefatigue training. Instead of extending the exercise set with a few reduced-resistance repetitions, prefatigue training essentially extends the exercise set with an immediate second exercise. The first exercise fatigues the target muscles with a single-muscle exercise, such as 10 leg extensions for the quadriceps. The second exercise further stimulates the target muscles with a multiple-muscle exercise such as 5 leg presses for the quadriceps, hamstrings, and gluteals. The fresh hamstrings and gluteal muscles assist the prefatigued quadriceps in performing a few leg presses, thereby pushing the quadriceps muscles to a deeper level of fatigue and providing a greater stimulus for strength development. In addition to being effective and efficient, prefatigue training uses two different exercises for the target muscle group, making this a more interesting and productive high-intensity training technique. This is because each exercise activates different force-producing fibers in the target muscles, thereby providing a more comprehensive conditioning effect.

Whether you perform the high-load, high-volume advanced training programs or the high-intensity, low-volume advanced training protocols, you should attain progressive gains in strength. Our exercise participants have had excellent results with both training procedures, so your workout selection is essentially a matter of personal preference. Just be sure to follow the principles of resistance training (e.g., overload, progression, recovery) and the exercise guidelines (e.g., speed, range, breathing) for safe and productive strength training sessions.

PROTOCOLS FOR ADVANCED STRENGTH TRAINING

The protocols for advanced strength training are presented for machine exercises; free-weight exercises; and body-weight, exercise ball, and resistance band training exercises. Programs 10.1, 10.3, and 10.5 require multiple set training and longer exercise sessions. These training programs involve higher-load and higher-volume exercise protocols. Programs 10.2, 10.4, and 10.6 require single-set training and shorter exercise sessions. These training programs involve lower-load and lower-volume exercise protocols but provide high-intensity workout sessions.

PROGRAM 10.1: HIGH LOAD

Program 10.1 is a machine workout that uses 12 basic exercises that train the most important major muscle groups. The first leg exercise is a linear action (straight movement) that works the muscles of the front thigh, rear thigh, and hip. The next two leg exercises are rotary actions (curved movements) that target the muscles of the inner thigh and outer thigh. The four upper-body exercises are linear actions that involved two or more major muscle groups concurrently and are arranged in an alternating push–pull sequence. The two arm exercises also address opposing muscle groups. The last three exercises are rotary actions that focus on the muscles of the midsection. You will note that the chest press (an upper-body pushing exercise) is followed by the seated row (an upper-body pulling exercise); the shoulder press (an upper-body pushing exercise) is paired with the pulldown (an upper-body pulling exercise). The triceps extension (muscles on the rear of the arm) is followed by the biceps curl (muscles on the front of the arm). Likewise, the abdominal exercise is followed by the low back exercise, and the oblique muscles are trained in pairs in both rotational directions. Alternating exercises for opposing muscle groups is an effective means of obtaining balanced strength development.

Program 10.1 is a multiple-set training protocol that uses progressively higher loads (percentages of maximum resistance) in successive exercise sets. For example, if you perform two exercise sets, the first set should use a load that you can lift about 12 repetitions at approximately 70 percent of maximum resistance. The second set should use a load that you can lift about 8 repetitions at approximately 80 percent of maximum resistance. If you choose to do three sets of each exercise, the third set should use a load that you can lift about 4 repetitions at approximately 90 percent of maximum resistance. This is a pyramid-style protocol in which successive sets are performed with higher loads and few repetitions. We refer to this exercise program as high-load training.

If you perform two sets of each exercise, with 90-second recovery periods, program 10.1 should take about 1 hour. Adding a third set of each exercise will extend your training time to approximately 90 minutes. The table presents the program 10.1 exercise sequence and performance information on training loads, repetitions, sets, repetition speed, and recovery periods.

Machine Training

Program 10.1—Machine Training (High Load)

Exercise	Muscle group	Page #
1. Leg press	Quadriceps, hamstrings, gluteals	62
2. Hip adduction	Hip adductors	64
3. Hip abduction	Hip abductors	65
4. Chest press	Pectoralis major, triceps, anterior deltoids	71
5. Seated row	Latissimus dorsi, middle trapezius, rhomboids, biceps, posterior deltoids, teres major	79
6. Shoulder press	Deltoids, triceps, upper trapezius	74
7. Lat pulldown	Latissimus dorsi, biceps, teres major	78
8. Triceps extension	Triceps	85
9. Biceps curl	Biceps	84
10. Abdominal flexion	Core: rectus abdominis	68
11. Low back extension	Core: erector spinae	67
12. Rotary torso	Core: external obliques, internal obliques, rectus abdominis	69

Training load	Repetitions	Sets	Repetition speed	Recovery time
70-90% max	4-12	2-3*	4-6 sec	90-120 sec

*If 2 sets: Set 1: 70% max × 12 reps.
Set 2: 80% max × 8 reps.
If 3 sets: Set 1: 70% max × 12 reps.
Set 2: 80% max × 8 reps.
Set 3: 90% max × 4 reps.

PROGRAM 10.2: HIGH INTENSITY

Program 10.2 is a high-intensity workout with 12 exercises that address most of the major muscle groups. This comprehensive strength training program includes four paired exercises and four independent exercises. To make this workout more challenging, you perform paired exercises for the muscles of the thigh, chest, upper back, and shoulder. In the thigh paired exercises, the first exercise is a rotary movement (leg curl) that targets the hamstring muscles. The second exercise is a linear movement (leg press) that works the same (prefatigued) hamstring muscles with assistance from fresh (nonfatigued) quadriceps and gluteus maximus muscles. In the chest paired exercises, the first exercise is a rotary movement (chest crossover) that works the target muscle group (pectoralis major). The second exercise is a linear movement (chest press) that also works the same (prefatigued) pectoralis major muscles with assistance from fresh (nonfatigued) triceps muscles. In the upper-back paired exercises, the first exercise is a rotary movement (pullover) that works the target muscle group (latissimus dorsi). The second exercise is a linear movement (lat pulldown) that challenges the same (prefatigued) latissimus dorsi muscles with assistance from fresh (nonfatigued) biceps muscles. In the shoulder paired exercise, the first exercise is a rotary movement (lateral raise) that addresses the target muscle group (deltoids). The second exercise is a linear movement (shoulder press) that works the same (prefatigued) deltoid muscles with help from fresh (nonfatigued) triceps muscles. This type of training, sometimes referred to as prefatigue training, is most effective with relatively short rests (15 seconds) between the paired exercises. Perform the exercises in the recommended order (rotary followed by linear) for best results.

Three of the exercises are performed with a different high-intensity protocol known as breakdown training. This technique involves two successive sets of the same exercise with only 5 seconds rest between sets. The first set is performed with a load that can be lifted for 8 to 12 repetitions. The second set is completed with approximately 20 percent less resistance for as many good repetitions as possible. For example, if you do 10 biceps curls to muscle fatigue with 50 pounds, you immediately reduce the resistance to 40 pounds and perform as many additional repetitions as possible (typically 4 to 6). Because of the high level of muscle fatigue caused by these extended exercise sets, you should find breakdown training to be a productive protocol for enhancing your muscle development.

Because of the relatively brief recovery periods inherent in high-intensity training, this exercise protocol should take less than 30 minutes. The table presents the program 10.2 exercise sequence and performance information on training loads, repetitions, sets, repetition speed, and recovery periods.

Machine Training

Program 10.2—Machine Training (High Intensity)

Exercise	Muscle group	Page #
1. Leg curl (P-1)	Hamstrings	61
2. Leg press (P-1)	Quadriceps, hamstrings, gluteals	62
3. Chest crossover (P-2)	Pectoralis major, anterior deltoids	70
4. Chest press (P-2)	Pectoralis major, anterior deltoids, triceps	71
5. Pullover (P-3)	Latissimus dorsi, teres major, triceps	76
6. Lat pulldown (P-3)	Latissimus dorsi, biceps, teres major	78
7. Lateral raise (P-4)	Deltoids	73
8. Shoulder press (P-4)	Deltoids, triceps, upper trapezius	74
9. Biceps curl (B)	Biceps	84
10. Triceps extension (B)	Triceps	85
11. Abdominal flexion (B)	Core: rectus abdominis	68
12. Low back extension	Core: erector spinae	67

Training load	Repetitions	Sets	Repetition speed	Recovery time
70-80% max	8-12	1 (modified)	4-6 sec	• 60-90 sec between exercises for different muscle groups • 15 sec between paired exercises for the same muscle groups • 5 sec between loads in breakdown training

P= Paired exercises
B = Breakdown training

PROGRAM 10.3: HIGH LOAD

Program 10.3 is a free-weight workout that features 12 exercises that address most of the major muscle groups. The first leg exercise is a linear barbell action that works the muscles of the front thigh, rear thigh, and hip. The second leg exercise is a linear dumbbell action that also uses the muscles of the front thigh, rear thigh, and hip in a different movement pattern. The third leg exercise is a linear dumbbell action that targets the calf muscles in the lower leg. The next five exercises involve the key upper-body muscles in an alternating manner. The bench press (an upper-body pushing exercise) is followed by the one-arm row (an upper-body pulling exercise). Likewise, the incline press (an upper-body pushing exercise) is followed by the pullover (an upper-body pulling exercise). The final upper-body exercise works the shoulder and neck muscles. The next two exercises are rotary actions for the upper arms, with the dumbbell curl for the biceps muscles followed by the dumbbell extension for the triceps muscles. The final two exercises in this training protocol are rotary movements for the front core (abdominal muscles) and rear core (low back muscles). This protocol fosters balanced muscle development and sequences the exercises from larger muscle groups to smaller muscle groups for a more effective training response.

Program 10.3 is a multiple-set training protocol that uses progressively higher loads (percentages of maximum resistance) in successive exercise sets. For example, if you perform two exercise sets, the first set should use a load that you can lift about 12 repetitions at approximately 70 percent of maximum resistance. The second set should use a load that you can lift about 8 repetitions at approximately 80 percent of maximum resistance. If you choose to do three sets of each exercise, the third set should use a load that you can lift about 4 repetitions at approximately 90 percent of maximum resistance. This is a pyramid-style training protocol in which successive sets are performed with higher loads and fewer repetitions. We refer to this exercise program simply as high-load training. Be sure to take 90 to 120 seconds of recovery time between the progressively heavier exercise sets.

If you perform two sets of each exercise, with 90-second recovery periods, program 10.3 should require about 1 hour. Adding a third set of each exercise will extend your training time to approximately 90 minutes. The table presents the program 10.3 exercise sequence and performance information on training loads, repetitions, sets, repetition speed, and recovery periods.

Program 10.3—Free-Weight Training (High Load)

Exercise	Muscle group	Page #
1. Barbell squat	Quadriceps, hamstrings, gluteals	94
2. Dumbbell lunge*	Quadriceps, hamstrings, gluteals	97
3. Dumbbell heel raise*	Gastrocnemius, soleus	98
4. Barbell bench press	Pectoralis major, anterior deltoids, triceps	112
5. Dumbbell one-arm row*	Latissimus dorsi, posterior deltoids, biceps, middle trapezius, rhomboids, teres major	126
6. Barbell incline press	Pectoralis major, anterior deltoids, triceps	114
7. Dumbbell pullover	Latissimus dorsi, triceps, teres major	124
8. Dumbbell alternating shoulder press	Deltoids, triceps, upper trapezius	120
9. Preacher curl	Biceps	133
10. Dumbbell overhead triceps extension	Triceps	135
11. Body-weight twisting trunk curl**	Core: rectus abdominis, external obliques, internal obliques, hip flexors, rectus femoris	152
12. Body-weight trunk extension**	Core: erector spinae	150

Training load	Repetitions	Sets	Repetition speed	Recovery time
70-90% max	4-12	2-3***	4-6 sec	90-120 sec

*May also be performed with kettlebells.

**Body-weight exercises: As many repetitions as necessary to fatigue the target muscles.

***If 2 sets: Set 1: 70% max x 12 reps.

Set 2: 80% max × 8 reps.

If 3 sets: Set 1: 70% max × 12 reps.

Set 2: 80% max × 8 reps.

Set 3: 90% max × 4 reps.

PROGRAM 10.4: HIGH INTENSITY

Program 10.4 is a high-intensity workout with 12 exercises that collectively train most of the major muscle groups. This well-balanced strength training program features eight paired exercises and four independent exercises. To make this workout more productive, you need to perform paired exercises for the muscles of the thigh, chest, upper back, and shoulder. In the paired exercises for the thigh, the first exercise is a barbell (linear) movement for the quadriceps, hamstrings, and gluteal muscles, and the following exercise is a dumbbell (linear) movement to further stress the same muscle groups. In the paired exercises for the chest, the first exercise is a rotary movement (dumbbell chest fly) that addresses the target muscle group (pectoralis major). The second exercise is a linear movement (barbell bench press) that hits the same (prefatigued) pectoralis major muscles with assistance from (nonfatigued) triceps muscles. In the upper-back paired exercises, the first exercise is a rotary movement (dumbbell pullover) that works the target muscle group (latissimus dorsi). The second exercise is a linear movement (dumbbell one-arm row) that challenges the same (prefatigued) latissimus dorsi muscles with help from fresh (nonfatigued) biceps muscles. In the shoulder paired exercises, the first exercise is a rotary movement (dumbbell lateral raise) that addresses the target muscle group (deltoids). The second exercise is a linear movement (dumbbell seated press) that works the same (prefatigued) deltoid muscles with assistance from fresh (nonfatigued) triceps muscles. This type of training, sometimes referred to as prefatigue training, is most effective with relatively short rests (15 seconds) between the paired exercises. Perform the exercises in the prescribed order (rotary followed by linear) for best results.

Two of the program 10.4 exercises are performed with another high-intensity protocol known as breakdown training. This technique involves two successive sets of the same exercise with only 5 seconds of rest between sets. The first set is performed with a load that can be lifted 8 to 12 repetitions. The next set is completed with approximately 20 percent less resistance for as many good repetitions as possible. For example, if you do 10 dumbbell incline curls to muscle fatigue with 25-pound dumbbells, you immediately switch to 20-pound dumbbells and perform as many additional repetitions as possible (typically 4 to 6 reps). Because of the high level of muscle fatigue caused by the successive exercise sets, you should find breakdown training to be a productive protocol for enhancing your muscle development.

Because of the relatively brief recovery periods, the program 10.4 training session should take less than 30 minutes. The table presents the program 10.4 exercise sequence and performance information on training loads, repetitions, sets, repetition speed, and recovery periods.

Program 10.4—Free-Weight Training (High Intensity)

Exercise	Muscle group	Page #
1. Barbell squat (P-2)	Quadriceps, hamstrings, gluteals	92
2. Dumbbell step-up (P-1)	Quadriceps, hamstrings, gluteals	96
3. Dumbbell chest fly (P-2)	Pectoralis major, anterior deltoids, serratus anterior	109
4. Barbell bench press (P-1)	Pectoralis major, anterior deltoids, triceps	112
5. Dumbbell pullover (P-2)	Latissimus dorsi, triceps, teres major	124
6. Dumbbell one-arm row (P-1)	Latissimus dorsi, posterior deltoids, biceps, middle trapezius, rhomboids, teres major	126
7. Dumbbell lateral raise (P-2)	Deltoids	118
8. Dumbbell seated press (P-1)	Deltoids, triceps, upper trapezius	119
9. Dumbbell incline curl (B-3,1)	Biceps	132
10. Dumbbell lying triceps extension (B-3,1)	Triceps	136
11. Body-weight twisting trunk curl (1)	Core: rectus abdominis, external obliques, internal obliques, hip flexors, rectus femoris	152
12. Body-weight trunk extension**	Core: erector spinae	150

Training load	Repetitions	Sets	Repetition speed	Recovery time
70-80% max	8-12	1 (modified)	4-6 sec	• 60-90 sec between exercises for different muscle groups • 15 sec between paired exercises for the same muscle groups • 5 sec between loads in breakdown training

P = Paired exercises
B = Breakdown training
*May also be performed using kettlebells.
**Body-weight exercises: As many repetitions as possible to fatigue the target muscles.

PROGRAM 10.5: HIGH LOAD

Program 10.5 is a resistance band workout that has nine basic exercises that address most of your major muscle groups. The first exercise is a linear movement that works the muscles of the front thigh, rear thigh, and hip. The next six exercises are alternating pushing and pulling movements for the muscles of the upper body and arms. The chest press is followed by the seated row for the opposing upper-back muscles. The next two exercises work the shoulder muscles, the first with assistance from the triceps muscles and the second with assistance from the biceps muscles. The two rotary arm exercises target the triceps muscles followed by the biceps muscles. The final two exercises in this program use body-weight resistance to address the front core (abdominal muscles) and rear core (low back muscles). This protocol is a balanced workout and sequences the exercise from larger muscle groups to smaller muscle groups for a more productive training response.

Like program 10.1 and program 10.3, this protocol provides multiple-set training that uses progressively higher loads (percentages of maximum resistance) in successive exercise sets. For example, if you perform two exercise sets, the first set should use a band that enables you to complete about 12 repetitions at approximately 70 percent of maximum resistance. The second set should use a thicker or stronger band that enables you to complete about 8 repetitions at approximately 80 percent of maximum resistance. If you choose to do three sets of each exercise, the third set should use an even stronger band that enables you to perform about 4 repetitions at approximately 90 percent of maximum resistance. This is a pyramid-style training protocol in which successive sets are performed with higher loads and fewer repetitions. We refer to this exercise program simply as high-load training. Be sure to take 90 to 120 seconds of recovery time between the progressively heavier exercise sets.

If you complete two sets of each exercise, with 90-second recovery periods, you should be capable of completing program 10.5 in 45 minutes. If you add a third set of each exercise, your training session should take 65 to 70 minutes. The table presents the program 10.5 exercise sequence and performance information on training resistance, repetitions, sets, repetition speed, and recovery periods.

Program 10.5—Resistance Band Training (High Load)

Exercise	Muscle group	Page #
1. Resistance band squat	Quadriceps, hamstrings, gluteals	148
2. Resistance band chest press	Pectoralis major, anterior deltoids, triceps	159
3. Resistance band seated row	Latissimus dorsi, posterior deltoids, biceps, middle trapezius, rhomboids, teres major	168
4. Resistance band seated press	Deltoids, triceps, upper trapezius	164
5. Resistance band upright row	Deltoids, biceps, upper trapezius	167
6. Resistance band one-arm triceps extension	Triceps	172
7. Resistance band biceps curl	Biceps	170
8. Body-weight twisting trunk curl*	Core: rectus abdominis, external obliques, internal obliques, hip flexors, rectus femoris	152
9. Body-weight trunk extension*	Core: erector spinae	150

Training load	Repetitions	Sets	Repetition speed	Recovery time
60-90% max	4-12	2-3**	4-6 sec	90-120 sec

*Body-weight exercises: As many repetitions as necessary to fatigue the target muscles.

**If 2 sets: Set 1: 70% max × 12 reps.

Set 2: 80% max × 8 reps.

If 3 sets: Set 1: 70% max × 12 reps.

Set 2: 80% max × 8 reps.

Set 3: 90% max × 4 reps.

PROGRAM 10.6: HIGH INTENSITY

Program 10.6 is an advanced strength training program that uses body-weight resistance in a high-intensity exercise protocol. The 11 exercises that make up this program address most of the major muscle groups. Four are performed with an exercise ball, three may be performed with or without an exercise ball, and four are performed with body weight only. The wall squat, leg lift, and heel-pull exercises for the hip and thigh muscles are executed with an appropriately sized exercise ball, as is the walk-out exercise for the upper-body pushing muscles. The push-up (upper-body muscles), trunk curl (abdominal muscles), and trunk extension (low back muscles) may be executed with an exercise ball for increased core involvement, if desired. The bar dip, chin-up, push-up, bench dip, and walk-out work the upper-body muscles, whereas the trunk curl, trunk extension, and twisting trunk curl address the core musculature.

When using external resistance (machines, free weights, resistance bands), you can pair rotary exercises and linear exercises for a productive prefatigue training effect. This is not easily accomplished with internal (body weight) resistance because the majority of body-weight exercises are linear movements. Likewise, with external resistance you can reduce the load at the point of momentary muscle fatigue for a beneficial breakdown training effect. However, this is difficult to do when using a fixed body-weight resistance. Consequently, we recommend a somewhat different approach for increasing the intensity of body-weight training.

You should perform the advanced body-weight, exercise ball, and resistance band training exercises in the same manner as you did in the basic training program—that is, as many perfect form repetitions as possible to the point of momentary muscle fatigue. After a very brief rest period (5 seconds), you should perform as many additional repetitions as possible using only the first half of the range of motion. This is a variation of the breakdown training technique, but instead of reducing the resistance as with external loading, you reduce the range of motion to enable a few postfatigue repetitions. For example, if you complete 8 full-range chin-ups to muscle fatigue (chin over bar), rest 5 seconds, then perform as many half-range chin-ups as possible (chin halfway to bar).

This high-intensity training technique should work well with the body-weight leg exercises (wall squat, leg lift, heel pull) and with the body-weight upper-body exercises (bar dip, chin-up, push-up, bench dip, and walk-out). It may be a little more challenging to implement this training procedure with the body-weight core exercises (trunk curl, trunk extension, twisting trunk curl), but you should have similar effects.

Because of the relatively brief recovery periods, the extended-set body-weight and exercise ball training program should take 22 to 33 minutes. The table presents the program 10.6 exercise sequence and performance information on training loads, repetitions, sets, repetition speed, and recovery periods.

Body-Weight and Exercise Ball Training

Program 10.6—Body-Weight and Exercise Ball Training (High Intensity)

Exercise	Muscle group	Page #
1. Wall squat*	Quadriceps, hamstrings, gluteals	144
2. Leg lift*	Quadriceps, hip flexors, rectus abdominis	146
3. Heel pull*	Hamstrings, hip flexors	145
4. Bar dip	Pectoralis major, anterior deltoids, triceps	161
5. Chin-up	Latissimus dorsi, biceps, teres major, posterior deltoids	166
6. Push-up*	Pectoralis major, anterior deltoids, triceps, rectus abdominis	160
7. Trunk curl*	Core: rectus abdominis	154
8. Bench dip	Triceps, pectoralis major, anterior deltoids	171
9. Trunk extension*	Core: erector spinae	150
10. Walk-out*	Triceps, pectoralis major, anterior deltoids	174
11. Twisting trunk curl	Core: rectus abdominis, external obliques, internal obliques, hip flexors, rectus femoris	152

Training load	Repetitions	Sets	Repetition speed	Recovery time
Body weight	As many as necessary to fatigue the target muscles	1 (modified)	4-6 sec	60-90 sec

*May be performed with exercise ball.

CONTINUATION OF TRAINING PROGRAMS

Congratulations on completing at least one of the advanced training programs presented in this chapter. At this point you may consider continuing your favorite program with minor modifications, such as changing some of the training exercises or the relationship between resistance and repetitions. You may also consider trying one of the other advanced training programs. For example, if you are currently doing a high-intensity training program, you may want to try a high-load training program or vice versa. Just be sure that whatever training protocol you select, you train your muscles to the point of muscle fatigue within the recommended repetition range (4 to 16 reps) with the appropriate exercise resistance (60 to 90 percent of maximum load). If you apply the training principles presented in this book, you should make continued progress toward your potential for muscular development.

11

Sport-Specific Training Programs

Many past-50 exercisers, including the authors, participate in a variety of sports and athletic activities. If you are like us, you take sport performance seriously and strive to do your best in every athletic endeavor. Although some senior athletes still compete in team sports such as soccer, ice hockey, basketball, and softball, most pursue individual or partner activities. This chapter presents specific strength training programs for enhancing your performance in the recreational physical activities that we believe are the most popular: running, cycling, swimming, skiing, tennis, and golf.

We take a twofold approach to strength training for improved sport conditioning. The first is to help you avoid the sport-related injuries typically associated with disproportionate strength and muscular imbalances, and the second is to provide you with exercises that strengthen the muscles that are most involved in your sport. Concerning this first objective, which is our primary focus, sprinting tends to strengthen the quadriceps muscles of the front of the thigh more than the hamstring muscles of the rear thigh. If the quadriceps muscles become disproportionately stronger than the opposing hamstring muscles, the chances of injuring the hamstrings increase. Conversely, distance running tends to strengthen the hamstring muscles more than the quadriceps muscles, increasing the likelihood that the quadriceps will become injured. Therefore, we encourage sprinters to include hamstring strengthening and stretching exercises in their workouts to reduce the risk of hamstring injuries, and we encourage distance runners to perform quadriceps strengthening and stretching exercises to lower the risk of injuring these muscles.

The calf muscles (gastrocnemius and soleus) are used extensively in running, too. Because of their involvement in every running stride, many people think that runners should focus their training on strengthening calf muscles. Indeed they should, but it is also important to strengthen the weaker counterpart, the shin muscles (anterior tibialis). If you strengthen only the larger and stronger calf muscles, they will eventually overpower the smaller and weaker shin muscles, which may lead to shin splints, stress fractures, and Achilles tendon problems. With this in mind, we recommend that runners always conclude strength training workouts with a set of weighted toe raises to strengthen the shin muscles and maintain muscular balance in the lower-leg musculature.

Training the muscles that are most prominent (prime movers) in a sport is important because it strengthens these muscles and increases performance power.

Success in most sports is ultimately related to performance power, which is the product of muscle force and movement speed.

Performance power = muscle force × movement speed

Increasing your movement speed involves complex neuromuscular phenomena and technical training programs that are beyond the scope of this book. Increasing your muscles' force, on the other hand, is a relatively simple process that is best accomplished by implementing the strength training principles, protocols, and procedures presented in the previous chapters. As you increase your strength, you automatically develop the tools to improve your ability to increase muscle force and produce more power.

It is necessary to strengthen and stretch the muscles that are less involved in a sport in order to reduce the risk of injury, and it is also necessary to strengthen and stretch the prime mover muscles in order to increase power production. It is therefore important to follow a sensible strength training program that works all of your major muscle groups. This will help you avoid injury and improve your overall sport performance.

For example, in our golf studies (Westcott, Dolan, and Cavicchi 1996), the relatively brief but comprehensive approach taken to overall muscle conditioning produced many positive outcomes, both expected and unexpected. In addition to increasing muscular strength, performance power, and club-head speed, the golfers found that they could play golf more frequently and for longer durations without fatigue. Best of all, none of the golf conditioning participants (including those who had been injured previously) reported a golf-related injury as long as they continued their strength training program.

In this chapter we present specific strength training programs for the sports of running, cycling, swimming, skiing, tennis, and golf. Although the exercises and training protocols are different for each activity, the programs work all of the major muscle groups in the manner most appropriate for ensuring overall strength, muscle balance, and power enhancement. You will learn how the major muscles are involved in each athletic event and how to train them properly for integrated strength development and improved sport performance.

STRENGTH TRAINING FOR RUNNERS

Distance running is a great sport that millions of competitive and recreational athletes enjoy at a variety of levels. Whether you prefer to jog a couple of miles through the neighborhood or are training to complete a marathon, distance running is an efficient means of aerobic conditioning. Unfortunately, distance running is considerably less beneficial for your musculoskeletal system, and injury rates among runners are extremely high. The relatively new field of sports medicine was in large part a response to the large number of running-related injuries that accompanied the running revolution of the 1970s.

Running involves an incredible amount of contact, but it is with road surfaces rather than other athletes. Every running stride places about three times the weight of your body on your feet, ankles, knees, and hip joints. These landing forces also stress your low back muscles and joints. The repetitive pounding causes micro-trauma to the shock-absorbing tissues. Under ideal conditions, these tissues recover completely within 24 hours. However, numerous factors may interfere with normal recovery processes, eventually resulting in weakened and injury-prone tissues. Factors such as longer running sessions, faster running paces, shorter recovery periods between workouts, downhill running, running on hard surfaces, frequent racing, poor nutritional habits, undesirable changes in sleeping patterns, and poor-quality shoes might singularly, or in combination, compromise your recovery from training and lead to injury.

Of course, you can take steps to reduce the amount of tissue trauma and decrease your risk of running-related injuries. Such precautions include gradually increasing training paces and distances, selecting running routes or courses on soft surfaces and level terrain, competing in fewer races, and paying careful attention to proper nutrition and sleep. The importance of obtaining guidance when selecting running shoes cannot be overemphasized.

However, one of the most effective means of minimizing tissue trauma is to develop stronger muscles, tendons, fascia, ligaments, and bones. This is the primary reason that every runner should engage in a regular strength training program. Consider the results of our four-year strength training project with the Notre Dame High School (Hingham, Massachusetts) girls' cross country and track teams (Westcott 1995). In this study, 30 distance runners participated in a basic and brief strength training program during the summer and winter months between their cross country and track seasons. Every Monday, Wednesday, and Friday, they performed a 30-minute strength training program that included exercises for each major muscle group. During each of these years, the cross country team won both the Massachusetts and New England championships. More important, during the same four years, only one runner had an injury that resulted in a missed practice session or meet.

Benefits of Strength Training

The Notre Dame runners realized that a sensible strength training program provided many benefits, including the following:

- Greater muscular strength
- Greater muscular endurance
- Greater joint flexibility
- Better body composition
- Reduced risk of injury
- Improved self-confidence
- Improved running economy

Although the first six strength training benefits should be self-explanatory, you might be intrigued by the improved running economy. In another research study at the University of New Hampshire (Johnston et al. 1995), the female cross country runners who participated in a strength training program had a significantly greater improvement in their running economy than their teammates who did not perform resistance exercise. They required 4 percent less oxygen at submaximal running speeds (7:30-, 7:00-, and 6:30-minute mile paces), meaning that they could run more efficiently and race faster than before.

Concerns of Runners

Despite the numerous advantages, the fact that so few runners regularly include strength training in their regimen continues to be a mystery. Perhaps the following four myths keep runners from strength training: increased body weight, decreased movement speed, less fluid running form, and fatigued muscles. Let's take a closer look at each of these issues.

Increased Body Weight   Very few people who regularly follow a strength training program have the genetic potential to develop large muscles. This is especially true for distance runners, who typically have ectomorphic (thin) physiques. Strength training will increase strength and endurance, but rarely will it result in significant weight gain or muscle enlargement.

Decreased Movement Speed   With respect to running speed, our studies and those of many others have shown that greater strength results in faster movement. We need only look at sprinters and middle-distance runners to realize that strength training has a positive impact on running speed because nearly all of these athletes perform regular strength training exercises.

Less Fluid Running Form   Running involves coordinated actions of the legs and the arms, and one cannot function without the other. Your right arm moves in opposition to your left leg, and your left arm moves in opposition to your right leg, each perfectly counterbalancing the other. That is why it is almost impossible to run fast and move your arms slowly or to move your arms fast and run slowly. By strengthening the upper-body muscles, you more effectively share the running effort between your arms and legs, resulting in more fluid running form.

Fatigued Muscles   Strenuous strength training sessions can cause a considerable amount of muscle fatigue that could adversely affect the quality and quantity of your runs. Therefore, relatively brief strength workouts that do not leave you exhausted are recommended. Remember that you are strength training to enhance your running performance, not to become a competitive weightlifter. Our program of strength training for runners requires just one or two sets of each exercise for the major muscle groups, which does not take much time or produce high levels of lasting fatigue. You may also choose to strength train only one or two days per week, which should make muscle fatigue even less likely.

Program Design for Runners

The strength training program followed by the Notre Dame athletes described earlier is a comprehensive conditioning program that addresses all of the major muscle groups. This program does not imitate specific running movements or emphasize specific running muscles; rather, it focuses on exercises that will develop balanced muscular strength to reduce the risk of injury and enhance running performance.

Some people believe that runners should complete numerous sets and many repetitions with light resistance to increase their endurance capacity. However, this is not the purpose of strength training. Remember that running is best for improving cardiorespiratory endurance and that strength training is best for increasing musculoskeletal strength.

Muscular strength is maximized by training with heavy loads (90 to 100 percent of maximum) for 1 to 5 repetitions. This type of strength training is characteristic of competitive weightlifters who typically have a high percentage of fast-twitch muscle fibers. However, heavy loads are not recommended for distance runners. Instead, distance runners, who usually have a higher percentage of slow-twitch muscle fibers, will benefit more by using lighter loads (60 to 70 percent of maximum resistance) that permit 12 to 16 repetitions per set. Whenever you can complete 16 repetitions using proper form in two successive workouts, increase the exercise load by 1 to 5 pounds (.45 to 2.5 kg). One to two sets of each exercise should be sufficient for producing desirable strength development.

Perform repetitions in a slow and controlled manner. Doing so will maximize muscle tension and minimize momentum, resulting in a better training effect and reducing the likelihood of injury. Each repetition should take 4 to 6 seconds (2 to 3 seconds for each lifting movement and 2 to 3 seconds for each lowering movement). We suggest that you train two or three times a week on nonconsecutive days. It is essential to breathe on every repetition because holding your breath can restrict blood flow and lead to undesirable increases in blood pressure. The recommended breathing pattern is to exhale during each lifting movement and to inhale during each lowering movement.

Strength Exercises for Runners

Runners can develop strength and endurance by performing a variety of exercises using machines, free weights, or body-weight and resistance band training. Tables 11.1 through 11.3 present our recommended strength training exercises for runners and the order in which they should be performed in the workout.

Even runners who train with machines, body weight, or resistance bands should consider concluding each exercise session with a set of weighted toe raises as shown in figure 11.1. This simple exercise strengthens the shin muscles (anterior tibialis) to maintain lower-leg muscle balance and reduce the risk of shin splints.

Summary for Running

The main objectives of a strength training program for runners are to decrease injuries while increasing muscular strength and running performance. The workout should be relatively short but reasonably strenuous. One set of 12 to 16 repetitions for each major muscle group will provide a safe and efficient exercise experience. Two or three training sessions per week are sufficient. Each workout should take 25 to 50 minutes, depending on the number of sets you perform.

Table 11.1 Strength Training for Runners: Machine Exercises

Exercise	Muscle group	Page #
1. Leg press	Quadriceps, hamstrings, gluteals	62
2. Heel raise	Gastrocnemius, soleus	66
3. Chest crossover	Pectoralis major, anterior deltoids, serratus anterior	70
4. Pullover	Latissimus dorsi, teres major	76
5. Lateral raise	Deltoids	73
6. Weight-assisted chin-up	Latissimus dorsi, biceps, teres major, posterior deltoids	80
7. Weight-assist bar dip	Pectoralis major, anterior deltoids, triceps	83
8. Abdominal flexion	Core: Rectus abdominis	68
9. Low back extension	Core: Erector spinae	67
10. Rotary torso	Core: Internal obliques, external obliques, rectus abdominis	69
11. Neck flexion and extension	Neck flexors, neck extensors	88, 89

Training load	Repetitions	Sets	Repetition speed	Recovery time
60-70% max	12-16	1-2	4-6 sec	60-90 sec

Table 11.2 Strength Training for Runners: Free-Weight Exercises

Exercise	Muscle group	Page #
1. Barbell or dumbbell squat	Quadriceps, hamstrings, gluteals	94, 92
2. Barbell or dumbbell heel raise	Gastrocnemius, soleus	100, 98
3. Barbell or dumbbell bench press	Pectoralis major, anterior deltoids, triceps	112, 110
4. Dumbbell double bent-over row	Latissimus dorsi, teres minor, rhomboids, middle trapezius, biceps, posterior deltoids	128
5. Dumbbell seated press	Deltoids, upper trapezius, triceps	119
6. Preacher curl	Biceps	133
7. Dumbbell lying triceps extension	Triceps	136
8. Body-weight trunk curl*	Core: Rectus abdominis	154
9. Body-weight trunk extension*	Core: Erector spinae	150
10. Body-weight twisting trunk curl*	Core: Rectus abdominis, internal obliques, external obliques, hip flexors, rectus femoris	152
11. Dumbbell or barbell shrug	Upper trapezius	141, 140
12. Weighted toe raise	Anterior tibialis	214

Training load	Repetitions	Sets	Repetition speed	Recovery time
60-70% max	12-16	1-2	4-6 sec	60-90 sec

*Body-weight exercises: As many repetitions as necessary to fatigue the target muscles.

Table 11.3 Strength Training for Runners: Body-Weight and Resistance Band Exercises

Exercise	Muscle group	Page #
1. Wall squat: exercise ball*	Quadriceps, hamstrings, gluteals	144
2. Exercise ball heel pull*	Hamstrings, hip flexors	145
3. Exercise ball leg lift*	Quadriceps, hip flexors, rectus abdominis	146
4. Body-weight push-up*	Pectoralis major, anterior deltoids, triceps, rectus abdominis	160
5. Resistance band seated row	Latissimus dorsi, teres major, rhomboids, middle trapezius, biceps, posterior deltoids	168
6. Resistance band seated press	Deltoid, upper trapezius, triceps	164
7. Body-weight chin-up*	Latissimus dorsi, biceps, teres major, posterior deltoids	166
8. Body-weight bar dip*	Pectoralis major, anterior deltoids, triceps	161
9. Body-weight trunk curl*	Core: Rectus abdominis	154
10. Body-weight trunk extension*	Core: Erector spinae	150
11. Body-weight twisting trunk curl*	Core: Rectus abdominis, internal obliques, external obliques, hip flexors, rectus femoris	152
12. Resistance band shrug	Upper trapezius	175

Training load	Repetitions	Sets	Repetition speed	Recovery time
60-70% max	12-16	1-2	4-6 sec	60-90 sec

*Body-weight exercises: As many repetitions as necessary to fatigue the target muscles.

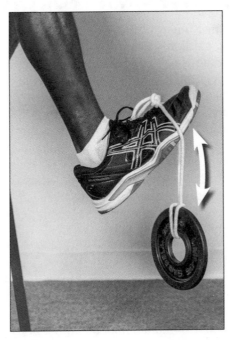

Figure 11.1 Weighted toe raise.

The key to productive strength training is proper exercise technique, which includes performing the exercises through the full range of motion and in a controlled manner. Be sure to eat enough calories to fuel your combined physical activities; include additional protein and lots of water. Finally, try to sleep at least eight hours nightly so that you enter every exercise session with energy and enthusiasm. After following these training recommendations for a couple of months, you could see your strength increase 40 to 60 percent and your running performance improve, too.

Exercise selection	Include appropriate exercises to cumulatively address all of the major muscle groups.
Training load	Use a training load that is 60 to 70 percent of maximum resistance.
Repetitions	Complete 12 to 16 controlled repetitions.
Progression	Increase the resistance by 5 percent when you can complete 16 repetitions during 2 successive sessions.
Sets	Complete 1 or 2 sets of each exercise.
Movement speed	Complete each movement at a moderate speed, taking 2 to 3 seconds to lift and 2 to 3 seconds to lower.
Movement range	Perform each exercise through a relatively full range of motion.
Training frequency	Complete 2 or 3 exercise sessions per week.

STRENGTH TRAINING FOR CYCLISTS

The bicycle is an extremely energy-efficient machine, and cycling is an excellent exercise for enhancing cardiorespiratory endurance. Like running, cycling uses the leg muscles to generate power. Unlike running, cycling does not generate landing forces to the feet, legs, and back, which reduces the risk of impact injuries. Nonetheless, cycling, like any repetitive-movement activity, stresses some muscles more than others, which may lead to overuse injuries.

Let's examine the major muscles involved in cycling. The power stroke in cycling is produced primarily by knee extension from contraction of the quadriceps muscles and hip extension from contraction of the hamstring muscles with assistance from the gluteal muscles of the buttocks. Lower-leg muscles also contribute. Cyclists use calf muscles while pushing on the pedals during ankle extension (gastrocnemius, soleus, plantaris) and engage the shin muscles when they pull against the pedal clips during ankle flexion (anterior tibialis).

Although the involvement of the thigh and lower-leg muscles in cycling is quite apparent, the role of the triceps, shoulders, and lower back muscles in maintaining the torso position is not. In addition, the upper-back and chest muscles provide stability for the upper-arm position, and forearm strength allows a firm grip on the handlebars. Proper positioning of the handlebars helps to evenly distribute the muscular requirements for maintaining the upper-body posture and delaying the onset of fatigue. The neck extensors help maintain the chin-up head position.

All of these muscles, therefore, require consideration when designing a strength training program for cyclists.

Like other athletes, you should strengthen all major muscle groups through a comprehensive strength training program. Train both the primary muscle groups and their opposing muscles in order to achieve balanced strength and muscular development across the various joint structures. Training only the primary muscles typically leads to overuse injuries because muscles on one side of a joint become much stronger than those on the other side, and the weaker musculature is eventually overpowered and damaged. This does not imply that you should train opposing muscle groups to equal strength levels. For example, the neck extensor muscles are inherently larger and stronger than the neck flexor muscles, so it would be nearly impossible to train both muscle groups to lift the same amount of resistance. The same is true of the muscles of the lower leg: The ankle extensor muscles in the calves are larger and stronger than the ankle flexor muscles in the shins; therefore, you should not try to train the extensor and flexor muscles to the same strength level. However, both sets of muscles should be addressed in a sensible strength training program for cyclists.

Program Design for Cyclists

The exercises in the strength training program for cyclists do not imitate specific movements or emphasize specific muscle groups; rather, they focus on resistance exercises that strengthen the muscle groups essential for improved cycling performance and reduced risk of injuries. Discussed next are our recommendations for range of motion and speed; loads, repetitions, and sets; frequency; progression; and breathing.

Range of Motion and Speed   Although cycling involves movements that take the legs through only the middle of the range of motion and requires static contractions of the upper-body muscles, you should perform strength exercises through the full range of motion. To improve cycling performance, it may be acceptable to perform part-range movements, but for safety purposes, you should perform full-range movements. Weakness at the ends of the range of motion might reduce joint integrity and increase the risk of injury.

Because the exercises in the strength training program for cyclists do not simulate cycling movements and because it would be difficult to perform leg strengthening exercises at the same rate you can pedal a bicycle—about 90 repetitions per minute—you should complete the exercises in a controlled manner at a moderate speed. This maximizes strength development and minimizes the risk of injury. Research has demonstrated excellent gains in strength from exercising at moderate movement speeds (Fiatarone et al. 1990; Nelson et al. 1994; Pratley et al. 1994; Westcott et al. 2009). We recommend 2 to 3 seconds for each lifting action and 2 to 3 seconds for each lowering action, or about 4 to 6 seconds per exercise repetition.

Loads, Repetitions, and Sets   To increase strength, the exercise resistance should be sufficient to fatigue the target muscles. Because cycling is an endurance activity, most cyclists should attain excellent strength gains by training with loads that result in 12 to 16 repetitions (equivalent to 60 to 70 percent of maximum resistance). Of course, this assumes training to the point of muscle fatigue on each exercise set. Cyclists require considerable time and energy to perform their daily training distance. Therefore, it is not advisable for cyclists to spend unnecessary time and energy in strength training. Fortunately, building muscular endurance and building muscular strength are complementary activities. That is, the same exercise program that develops strength also increases muscular endurance. Research indicates that one or two sets of properly performed strength training exercise is sufficient for stimulating significant gains in strength and endurance (Starkey et al. 1996; Westcott, Greenberger, and Milius 1989). Therefore, you should start with one set of each exercise and add a second set as your muscular fitness improves, if you choose to do so.

For maximum benefit, you should perform each set of exercises to muscle fatigue or temporary muscle failure. This means that you exercise until your muscles cannot complete another repetition with proper form.

Frequency Research shows that two or three properly spaced training sessions per week are effective for improving muscular strength (Braith et al. 1989; DeMichele et al. 1997; Westcott et al. 2009). Cyclists who schedule two strength workouts per week invest a relatively small amount of time for relatively large improvements in strength and endurance. Research with adults over age 50 as well as with elderly individuals reveals an increase in muscular strength of approximately 50 percent after just two to three months of twice-a-week resistance training (Westcott, Dolan, and Cavicchi 1996; Westcott et al. 2009).

Progression We prefer a double-progressive system of strength development. Begin with a load that you can lift 12 times, and continue training with it until you can complete 16 repetitions. When you perform 16 repetitions on two successive occasions, increase the resistance by about 5 percent. Stay with this load until you can complete 16 repetitions, and then again increase the resistance by about 5 percent.

Breathing Remember to breathe throughout every repetition. Exhale during each lifting movement and inhale during each lowering movement.

Strength Exercises for Cyclists

Cyclists can develop strength and endurance by performing a variety of exercises using machines, free weights, or body-weight and resistance band training. Tables 11.4 through 11.6 present our recommended strength training exercises for cyclists and the order in which they should be performed in the workout.

Summary for Cycling

In our experience with cyclists and triathletes, stronger muscles lead to better cycling performance. Because every pedal revolution requires a certain percentage of maximum leg strength, more strength is of considerable advantage. After

Table 11.4 Strength Training for Cyclists: Machine Exercises

Exercise	Muscle group	Page #
1. Leg extension	Quadriceps	60
2. Leg curl	Hamstrings	61
3. Leg press	Quadriceps, hamstrings, gluteals	62
4. Chest crossover	Pectoralis major, anterior deltoids, serratus anterior	70
5. Chest press	Pectoralis major, anterior deltoids, triceps	71
6. Pullover	Latissimus dorsi, teres major, triceps	76
7. Seated row	Latissimus dorsi, teres major, rhomboids, middle trapezius, biceps, posterior deltoids	79
8. Lateral raise	Deltoids	73
9. Shoulder press	Deltoids, upper trapezius, triceps	74
10. Biceps curl	Biceps	84
11. Triceps extension	Triceps	85
12. Abdominal flexion	Core: Rectus abdominis	68
13. Low back extension	Core: Erector spinae	67
14. Neck flexion and extension	Neck flexors, neck extensors	88, 89

Training load	Repetitions	Sets	Repetition speed	Recovery time
60-70% max	12-16	1-2	4-6 sec	60-90 sec

Table 11.5 Strength Training for Cyclists: Free-Weight Exercises

Exercise	Muscle group	Page #
1. Barbell or dumbbell squat	Quadriceps, hamstrings, gluteals	94, 92
2. Dumbbell lunge	Quadriceps, hamstrings, gluteals	97
3. Barbell, dumbbell, or kettlebell heel raise	Gastrocnemius, soleus	100, 98
4. Dumbbell chest fly	Pectoralis major, anterior deltoids. serratus anterior	109
5. Barbell or dumbbell bench press	Pectoralis major, anterior deltoids, triceps	112, 110
6. Dumbbell pullover	Latissimus dorsi, teres major, triceps	124
7. Dumbbell double bent-over row	Latissimus dorsi, teres minor, rhomboids, middle trapezius, biceps	128
8. Dumbbell lateral raise	Deltoids	118
9. Dumbbell seated press	Deltoids, upper trapezius, triceps	119
10. Dumbbell curl	Biceps	130
11. Dumbbell lying triceps extension	Triceps	136
12. Body-weight trunk curl*	Core: Rectus abdominis	154
13. Body-weight trunk extension*	Core: Erector spinae	150
14. Barbell or dumbbell shrug	Upper trapezius	140, 141

Training load	Repetitions	Sets	Repetition speed	Recovery time
60-70% max	12-16	1-2	4-6 sec	60-90 sec

*Body-weight exercises: As many repetitions as necessary to fatigue all target muscles.

Table 11.6 Strength Training for Cyclists: Body-Weight and Resistance Band Exercises

Exercise	Muscle group	Page #
1. Resistance band squat	Quadriceps, hamstrings, gluteals	148
2. Exercise ball heel pull*	Hamstrings, hip flexors	145
3. Exercise ball leg lift*	Quadriceps, hip flexors, rectus abdominis	146
4. Body-weight push-up*	Pectoralis major, anterior deltoids, triceps, rectus abdominis	160
5. Resistance band chest press	Pectoralis major, anterior deltoids, triceps	159
6. Body-weight chin-up*	Latissimus dorsi, biceps	166
7. Resistance band seated row	Latissimus dorsi, teres major, rhomboids, middle trapezius, biceps, posterior deltoids	168
8. Resistance band seated press	Deltoids, upper trapezius, triceps	164
9. Body-weight trunk curl*	Core: Rectus abdominis	154
10. Body-weight trunk extension*	Core: Erector spinae	150
11. Resistance band shrug	Upper trapezius	175

Training load	Repetitions	Sets	Repetition speed	Recovery time
60-70% max	12-16	1-2	4-6 sec	60-90 sec

*Body-weight exercises: As many repetitions as necessary to fatigue all target muscles.

strength training, many cyclists are able to use higher gears at the same pedal frequency, thereby increasing their road speed. Be sure to eat enough calories to fuel your combined physical activities, consume sufficient protein, and drink lots of water. Finally, try to sleep at least eight hours nightly so that you enter every exercise session with energy and enthusiasm.

When developing a sensible strength training program, carefully consider the following exercise guidelines:

Exercise selection Include appropriate exercises to cumulatively address all of the major muscle groups.

Training load Use a training load that is 60 to 70 percent of maximum resistance.

Repetitions Complete 12 to 16 controlled repetitions.

Progression Increase the resistance by 5 percent when you can complete 16 repetitions during 2 successive sessions.

Sets Complete one set of each exercise.

Movement speed Complete each movement at a moderate speed, taking 2 to 3 seconds to lift and 2 to 3 seconds to lower.

Movement range Perform each exercise through a relatively full range of motion.

Training frequency Complete 2 or 3 exercise sessions per week.

STRENGTH TRAINING FOR SWIMMERS

Swimming has been called the perfect physical activity because it appears to address all of the body's major muscle groups. Indeed, swimming involves both the upper body and lower body through pulling movements of the arms and kicking actions of the legs. Nonetheless, some of the major muscle groups are used much more than others, thereby increasing the risk of overuse and imbalance injuries. For example, the upper-body muscles that pull the arms through the water work considerably harder than the opposing muscles that recover the arms through the air. Also, the leg muscles, which are continuously active, move through a relatively short and repetitive range of motion. This can lead to muscular imbalances. Because swimming is an aerobic activity, it is not a particularly good exercise for developing strength. However, increasing strength will significantly contribute to your success in swimming. Let's examine how strength training can enhance swimming performance as well as reduce injury potential.

Program Design for Swimmers

The recommended strength exercises for swimmers address the major muscle groups. The following guidelines for range of motion and speed; loads, repetitions, and sets; frequency; progression; and breathing should produce excellent results.

Range of Motion and Speed Although standard swimming strokes work the upper-body muscles through a fairly full range of motion, the kicking action of the legs uses only midrange movements. To avoid creating a muscular imbalance, perform exercises through a full range of motion but never to the point of discomfort. Also, move through a full range of motion in a slow and controlled manner. Quickly performed repetitions create momentum that might place excessive stress on muscles and joint structures.

Loads, Repetitions, and Sets Muscle strength is best developed by fatiguing the target muscles in the time boundaries of the anaerobic energy system, which typically requires 30 to 90 seconds. At a controlled movement speed of 4 to 6 seconds per repetition, a set of 8 to 12 repetitions can be completed in this time frame. Most people can perform 8 to 12 repetitions with 70 to 80 percent of their maximum resistance, which is a safe and productive load. Although periodically you may want to train with more or fewer repetitions, 8 to 12 repetitions are appropriate for most practical purposes.

Many studies show that the strength building benefits that are achieved in single-set training are similar to those achieved in multiple-set training (Starkey et al. 1996; Westcott, Greenberger, and Milius 1989). The number of sets you perform is largely a matter of personal preference and available time. You can achieve significant results by doing a warm-up set with 50 percent of the training load and then resting 60 seconds, then performing one or two sets of the exercise to momentary muscle fatigue with the training load. These training protocols are both effective and efficient.

Frequency Research reveals that two training sessions per week produce about the same strength as three training sessions per week, and for some, two days a week are preferable because they allow more time for recovery and muscle rebuilding (Braith et al. 1989; DeMichele et al. 1997; Westcott et al. 2009). Begin your workout with exercises for the larger muscle groups of the legs followed by the upper-body muscles, and finish with the muscles of the midsection and neck. Like the number of sets, the frequency of strength training is largely a matter of personal preference and available time.

Progression If you perform 8 to 12 repetitions per set, then you need a policy of sensible progression. Because muscular strength develops gradually, you should not increase the resistance more than 5 percent at a time. Continue lifting a given load until you can complete 12 repetitions with good form during two successive workouts. Then you can increase the resistance by 5 percent (usually 1 to 5 pounds, or .45 to 2.5 kg) in your next workout. This double-progressive system—first adding more repetitions, then adding a heavier load—is a safe and sound method for stimulating consistent gains in strength.

Breathing Breathe continuously during every training set. Try to exhale throughout each lifting movement and inhale throughout each lowering movement.

Strength Exercises for Swimmers

Swimmers can develop strength and endurance by performing a variety of exercises using machines, free weights, or body-weight and resistance band training. Tables 11.7 through 11.9 present our recommended strength training exercises for swimmers and the order in which they should be performed in the workout.

Table 11.7 Strength Training for Swimmers: Machine Exercises

Exercise	Muscle group	Page #
1. Leg extension	Quadriceps	60
2. Leg curl	Hamstrings	61
3. Leg press	Quadriceps, hamstrings, gluteals	62
4. Chest press	Pectoralis major, anterior deltoids, triceps	71
5. Pullover	Latissimus dorsi, teres major, triceps	76
6. Incline press	Pectoralis major, anterior deltoids, triceps	72
7. Lat pulldown	Latissimus dorsi, teres major, biceps	78
8. Shoulder press	Deltoids, upper trapezius, triceps	74
9. Seated row	Latissimus dorsi, teres major, rhomboids, middle trapezius, biceps, posterior deltoids	79
10. Abdominal flexion	Core: Rectus abdominis	68
11. Low back extension	Core: Erector spinae	67
12. Rotary torso	Core: Internal obliques, external obliques, rectus abdominis	69
13. Neck flexion and extension	Neck flexors, neck extensors	88, 89

Training load	Repetitions	Sets	Repetition speed	Recovery time
70-80% max	8-12	1-2	4-6 sec	60-90 sec

Table 11.8 Strength Training for Swimmers: Free-Weight Exercises

Exercise	Muscle group	Page #
1. Barbell or dumbbell squat	Quadriceps, hamstrings, gluteals	94, 92
2. Dumbbell step-up	Quadriceps, hamstrings, gluteals	96
3. Barbell or dumbbell bench press	Pectoralis major, anterior deltoids, triceps	112, 110
4. Dumbbell pullover	Latissimus dorsi, teres major, triceps	124
5. Barbell or dumbbell incline press	Pectoralis major, anterior deltoids, triceps	114, 116
6. Dumbbell double bent-over row	Latissimus dorsi, teres minor, rhomboids, middle trapezius, biceps, posterior deltoids	128
7. Dumbbell alternating shoulder press	Deltoids, upper trapezius, triceps	120
8. Dumbbell curl	Biceps	130
9. Dumbbell lying triceps extension	Triceps	136
10. Body-weight trunk curl*	Core: Rectus abdominis	154
11. Body-weight trunk extension*	Core: Erector spinae	150
12. Body-weight twisting trunk curl*	Core: Rectus abdominis, internal obliques, external obliques, hip flexors, rectus femoris	152
13. Barbell or dumbbell shrug	Upper trapezius	140, 141

Training load	Repetitions	Sets	Repetition speed	Recovery time
70-80% max	8-12	1-2	4-6 sec	60-90 sec

*Body-weight exercises: As many repetitions as necessary to fatigue the target muscles.

Table 11.9 Strength Training for Swimmers: Body-Weight and Resistance Band Exercises

Exercise	Muscle group	Page #
1. Wall squat: exercise ball*	Quadriceps, hamstrings, gluteals	144
2. Exercise ball heel pull*	Hamstrings, hip flexors	145
3. Exercise ball leg lift*	Quadriceps, hip flexors, rectus abdominis	146
4. Body-weight bar dip*	Pectoralis major, anterior deltoids, triceps	161
5. Body-weight chin-up*	Latissimus dorsi, biceps, teres major, posterior deltoids	166
6. Resistance band seated press	Deltoids, upper trapezius, triceps	164
7. Resistance band chest press	Pectoralis major, anterior deltoids, triceps	159
8. Resistance band seated row	Latissimus dorsi, teres major, rhomboids, middle trapezius, biceps, posterior deltoids	168
9. Body-weight push-up*	Pectoralis major, anterior deltoids, triceps, rectus abdominis	160
10. Resistance band biceps curl	Biceps	170
11. Body-weight trunk curl*	Core: Rectus abdominis	154
12. Body-weight trunk extension*	Core: Erector spinae	150
13. Body-weight twisting trunk curl*	Core: Rectus abdominis, internal obliques, external obliques, hip flexors, rectus femoris	152
14. Resistance band shrug	Upper trapezius	175

Training load	Repetitions	Sets	Repetition speed	Recovery time
70-80% max	8-12	1-2	4-6 sec	60-90 sec

*Body-weight exercises: As many repetitions as necessary to fatigue the target muscles.

Summary for Swimming

In our experience with swimmers, stronger muscles lead to better swimming performances. Because every swimming stroke and push off the wall requires a certain percentage of maximum arm and leg power, more muscular strength is a considerable advantage. After strength training, you should be able to perform at a higher strength level for a longer time. When developing a sensible swimming strength training program, consider the following exercise guidelines:

Exercise selection	Include appropriate exercises to cumulatively address all of the major muscle groups.
Training load	Use a training load that is about 70 to 80 percent of the maximum resistance.
Repetitions	Complete 8 to 12 controlled repetitions.
Progression	Increase the resistance by 5 percent when you can lift 12 repetitions during 2 successive sessions.
Sets	Complete 1 or 2 sets of each exercise.
Movement speed	Complete each movement at a moderate speed, taking 2 to 3 seconds to lift and 2 to 3 seconds to lower.
Movement range	Perform each exercise through a relatively full range of motion.
Training frequency	Complete 2 or 3 exercise sessions per week.

The strength training program for swimmers requires 25 to 50 minutes depending on the number of sets you perform. Although strength training should not interfere with swimming practice, it is probably best to schedule workouts on nonswimming days if possible. Be sure to eat enough calories to fuel your combined physical activities; include a little more protein and lots of water. Finally, try to sleep at least eight hours nightly so that you enter every exercise session with energy and enthusiasm.

STRENGTH TRAINING FOR SKIERS

In spite of the fact that chairlifts take you up the mountain, downhill skiing is a physically demanding activity. The body positions that provide the best combination of balance, stability, control, and speed are those that require relatively high levels of muscular strength. In addition to enhanced skiing performance, a strong musculoskeletal system is your best protection against the acute and overuse injuries that are all too common in this sport.

Although no one would argue the value of cardiorespiratory conditioning, clearly it is not the limiting factor in downhill skiing. And although a lack of joint flexibility may lead to performance limitations, excessive joint mobility is typically more harmful than helpful. The key to better skiing is greater muscular strength, pure and simple. For overall health and fitness, do your favorite endurance activities and stretching exercises. But for confidence and competence on the black diamond trails, do your strength training.

Downhill skiing is a power activity that emphasizes the anaerobic energy system. Forceful contractions of the quadriceps and hamstring muscles position the body to use the snow and gravity to best advantage. Be thankful for turns because they offer both challenge and change of position. You can't hold the power position for very long during a turn without causing formidable muscle fatigue; therefore, you must change your posture. This brief unloading phase provides momentary release and relief for the hard-working quadriceps and hamstrings. The turning action also activates the rotational muscles of the midsection and the lateral-movement muscles of the thighs. More specifically, smooth turns are closely related to strong external and internal oblique muscles that control midsection rotation and strong hip abductor and adductor muscles that shift the hips from side to side.

Although not as important for power production, the muscles of the shoulders, torso, and arms are responsible for effective pole plants and for safely absorbing impact during a fall. Other muscles that provide postural support and play a role in injury prevention are the low back and neck muscles. Finally, the anterior tibial muscles of the shin largely control the ankle joint during skiing movements. Although modern ski boots reduce ankle injuries, strong anterior tibial muscles are advantageous for better skiing performance and lower risk of injury.

Program Design for Skiers

A well-designed strength training program for skiers takes into consideration the number of repetitions to perform with a specific load, the number of training sessions per week, and guidelines for progressing to heavier loads. Because strength development is more closely related to intensity than to duration, you can achieve excellent results using relatively short workouts. The following guidelines for range of motion and speed; loads, repetitions, and sets; frequency; progression; and breathing should produce excellent results.

Range of Motion and Speed Strength is developed by exercising against resistance. Therefore, to develop strength throughout the entire range of a joint's movement, you must apply resistance during the full range, working the target muscle from the fully stretched position to the fully contracted position.

Slow strength training movements are more productive than fast strength training movements. This is because slow movement speeds produce more muscle force and muscle tension than fast movement speeds. Slower movement speeds also create less momentum, which focuses the effort on the target muscles. Because downhill skiing involves mostly eccentric muscle contractions, you should carefully control the lowering phase of each repetition. Our recommendation is 4- to 6-second repetitions with to 2 to 3 seconds for each lifting movement and 2 to 3 seconds for each lowering movement.

Loads, Repetitions, and Sets Muscular strength is best developed by fatiguing the target muscles, which in a typical strength training workout takes 30 to 90 seconds. At a controlled speed of 4 to 6 seconds per repetition, a set of 8 to 12 repetitions takes 35 to 75 seconds. Most people can perform 8 to 12 repetitions with 70 to 80 percent of their maximum resistance, which is safe and productive.

Although you may periodically want to train with more or fewer repetitions, 8 to 12 repetitions per set are appropriate for most purposes.

Many studies show that the strength benefits achieved in single-set training are similar to those achieved in multiple-set training (Starkey et al. 1996; Westcott, Greenberger, and Milius 1989). The number of sets you perform is largely a matter of personal preference and available time. The participants in our ski conditioning program have had excellent results by doing a warm-up set with 50 percent of their training load, resting 60 seconds, and then performing one set to momentary muscle fatigue with their training load. However, you may perform a second set of some or all of the recommended exercises if you would like. These training protocols are both effective and efficient.

Frequency Research reveals that two training sessions per week produce about the same muscle development as three training sessions per week (Braith et al. 1989; DeMichele et al. 1997; Westcott et al. 2009). For some people, two days a week is preferable because it allows more time for recovery and muscle remodeling. Because a gradual gain in strength is the major training objective, resist the temptation to do too much too soon. As with the number of sets, the frequency of strength training sessions is largely a matter of personal preference and available time.

Progression If you perform 8 to 12 repetitions per set, you need a sensible progression plan. Because muscular strength develops gradually, you should not increase the resistance more than 5 percent in any training session. Continue lifting a given load until you can complete 12 repetitions with good form for two successive workouts. Then increase the resistance by 5 percent (usually 1 to 5 pounds [.45 to 2.5 kg]) during your next workout. This double-progressive system—first adding more repetitions, then adding a heavier load—is a safe and sound method for stimulating consistent gains in strength.

Breathing Breathe on every repetition because holding your breath can lead to undesirable increases in blood pressure and restricted blood flow. Exhale during each lifting movement, and inhale during each lowering movement.

Strength Exercises for Skiers

Skiers can increase strength and endurance by performing a variety of exercises using machines, free weights, or body-weight and resistance band training. Tables 11.10 through 11.12 present our recommended strength training exercises for downhill skiers and the order in which they should be performed in the workout.

Summary for Skiing

Resistance exercise is effective for conditioning of downhill skiing. Be sure to eat enough calories to fuel your combined physical activities (strength training and skiing), including more protein and lots of water. Finally, try to sleep at least eight hours nightly so that you enter every exercise session with energy and enthusiasm.

Table 11.10 Strength Training for Skiers: Machine Exercises

Exercise	Muscle group	Page #
1. Leg extension	Quadriceps	60
2. Leg curl	Hamstrings	61
3. Hip adduction	Hip abductors	64
4. Hip abduction	Hip adductors	65
5. Leg press	Quadriceps, hamstrings, gluteals	62
6. Chest crossover	Pectoralis major, anterior deltoids, serratus anterior	70
7. Pullover	Latissimus dorsi, teres major, triceps	76
8. Lateral raise	Deltoids	73
9. Biceps curl	Biceps	84
10. Triceps extension	Triceps	85
11. Abdominal flexion	Core: Rectus abdominis	68
12. Low back extension	Core: Erector spinae	67
13. Rotary torso	Core: Rectus abdominis, internal obliques, external obliques	69
14. Neck flexion and extension	Neck flexors, neck extensors	89, 88

Training load	Repetitions	Sets	Repetition speed	Recovery time
70-80% max	8-12	1-2	4-6 sec	60-90 sec

Table 11.11 Strength Training for Skiers: Free-Weight Exercises

Exercise	Muscle group	Page #
1. Barbell or dumbbell squat	Quadriceps, hamstrings, gluteals	94, 92
2. Dumbbell lunge	Quadriceps, hamstrings, gluteals	97
3. Dumbbell step-up	Quadriceps, hamstrings, gluteals	96
4. Dumbbell chest fly	Pectoralis major, anterior deltoids, serratus anterior	109
5. Dumbbell pullover	Latissimus dorsi, teres major, triceps	124
6. Dumbbell lateral raise	Deltoids	118
7. Dumbbell curl	Biceps	130
8. Dumbbell overhead triceps extension	Triceps	135
9. Body-weight trunk curl*	Core: Rectus abdominis	154
10. Body-weight trunk extension*	Core: Erector spinae	150
11. Body-weight twisting trunk curl*	Core: Rectus abdominis, internal obliques, external obliques, hip flexors, rectus femoris	152
13. Dumbbell shrug	Upper trapezius	141

Training load	Repetitions	Sets	Repetition speed	Recovery time
70-80% max	8-12	1-2	4-6 sec	60-90 sec

*Body-weight exercises: As many repetitions as necessary to fatigue the target muscles.

Table 11.12   Strength Training for Skiers: Body-Weight and Resistance Band Exercises

Exercise	Muscle group	Page #
1. Wall squat: exercise ball*	Quadriceps, hamstrings, gluteals	144
2. Exercise ball heel pull*	Hamstrings, hip flexors	145
3. Exercise ball leg lift*	Quadriceps, hip flexors, rectus abdominis	146
4. Body-weight bench dip*	Pectoralis major, anterior deltoids, triceps	171
5. Resistance band seated row	Latissimus dorsi, teres major, rhomboids, middle trapezius, biceps, posterior deltoids	168
6. Resistance band seated press	Deltoids, upper trapezius, triceps	164
7. Body-weight trunk curl*	Core: Rectus abdominis	154
8. Body-weight trunk extension*	Core: Erector spinae	150
9. Body-weight twisting trunk curl*	Core: Rectus abdominis, internal obliques, external obliques, hip flexors, rectus femoris	152
10. Resistance band shrug	Upper trapezius	175

Training load	Repetitions	Sets	Repetition speed	Recovery time
70-80% max	8-12	1-2	4-6 sec	60-90 sec

*Body-weight exercises: As many repetitions as necessary to fatigue the target muscles.

When developing a sensible strength training program, carefully consider the following exercise guidelines:

Exercise selection	Include appropriate exercises to cumulatively address all of the major muscle groups.
Training load	Use a training load that is 70 to 80 percent of maximum resistance.
Repetitions	Complete 8 to 12 controlled repetitions.
Progression	Increase the resistance by 5 percent when you can complete 12 repetitions in 2 successive sessions.
Sets	Complete 1 or 2 sets of each exercise.
Movement speed	Complete each movement at a moderate speed, taking 2 to 3 seconds to lift and 2 to 3 seconds to lower.
Movement range	Perform each exercise through a relatively full range of motion.
Training frequency	Complete 2 or 3 exercise sessions per week.

STRENGTH TRAINING FOR TENNIS PLAYERS

Tennis requires excellent eye–hand coordination and agility and keen spatial awareness. In addition to the physical and mental challenge, a good singles match provides both anaerobic and aerobic conditioning. Although skill is essential for top-level tennis, technique development is easier if you are fit—which is also the critical factor for staying power during the second and third sets.

Fitness comes in many forms, and conditioning is specific to the type of training program you follow. For example, stretching exercises enhance joint flexibility, aerobic activity improves cardiorespiratory endurance, and strength training increases muscular strength. Certainly, all of these fitness components contribute to better tennis performance. However, if you choose to focus on only one area of physical conditioning for tennis, it should be strength training.

Specific Exercises for Tennis Players

Because playing tennis involves strenuous musculoskeletal activity in the legs, core, upper body, and arms, you should train all of the major muscle groups to ensure overall strength and balanced muscular development. This will enhance power and reduce the risk of injuries.

Shoulder Rotator Muscles   The rotator cuff consists of a group of muscles (supraspinatus, infraspinatus, teres minor, subscapularis) that surround and stabilize the shoulder joint. The shoulder rotator muscles lie beneath the large deltoid muscles and allow the arms to rotate into various positions. Rotating your arm backward, called external shoulder rotation, uses the teres minor and infraspinatus muscles. Rotating your arm forward, called internal shoulder rotation, involves the subscapularis muscles. Keeping the arm within the structure of the shoulder joint is the primary function of the supraspinatus muscle. Together, these four muscles surround the shoulder joint, providing both structural stability and the ability to produce powerful forehand, backhand, and serving movements.

The good news is that these four relatively small muscles respond well to strength training. The bad news is that most people do not perform specific exercises for the rotator cuff muscles. This is unfortunate because rotator cuff injuries occur frequently in tennis players and typically require a long recovery period. A well-designed strength training program should include at least one workout per week for the shoulder rotator muscles.

You may strengthen the typically weak external shoulder rotator muscles with dumbbells or resistance bands (figures 11.2 and 11.3). When using a dumbbell, position the upper

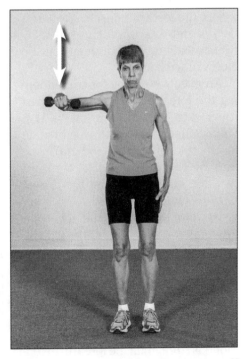

Figure 11.2   Strengthening the rotator cuff muscles with a dumbbell or weight plate.

arm and forearm at a right angle parallel to the floor, and maintain this upperarm position throughout the exercise. Slowly lift the dumbbell upward while maintaining the 90-degree elbow position (figure 11.2). Slowly lower the dumbbell to the starting position.

When using resistance bands, attach one end to a door at waist level, stand with your left side toward the door, keep your right elbow against your right side, and pull the band across your midsection using your right hand as shown in figure 11.3. Next, stand with your right side toward the door, keep your left elbow against your left side and pull the band across your midsection using your left hand. Tennis players should strengthen their rotator cuff muscles for improved performance and reduced risk of injury.

Forearm Muscles Because of the extensive wrist action required for tennis, the forearm muscles (forearm flexors and extensors) can be easily overstressed, leading to injury at the elbow or wrist joints.

An effective means for strengthening the forearm muscles is the wrist roller exercise shown in figure 11.4. Simply attach a 5-pound weight plate to one end of a 2-foot (60 cm) rope and tie the other end to a round wooden dowel. Holding the dowel in both hands, repeatedly flex your wrists clockwise to wind the rope around the dowel and lift the weight. When the weight touches the dowel, repeatedly extend your wrists counterclockwise to unwind the rope and lower the weight. The clockwise wrist motion strengthens the forearm flexor muscles, and counterclockwise wrist motions strengthen the forearm extensor muscles. Perform the wrist roller exercise at least once a week.

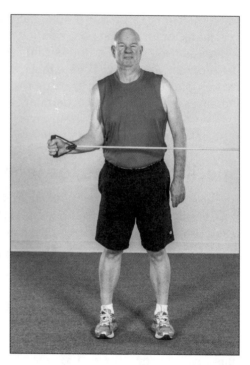

Figure 11.3 Using resistance bands to strengthen the rotator cuff muscles.

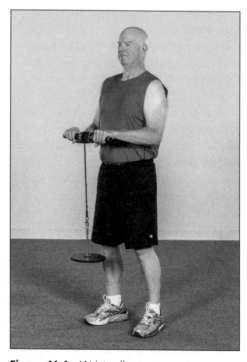

Figure 11.4 Wrist roller.

Program Design for Tennis Players

The exercises in the strength training program for tennis players do not imitate specific movements or emphasize particular muscles; rather, they focus on the exercises that strengthen all the muscle groups used in tennis. The following guidelines for range of motion and speed; loads, repetitions, and sets; frequency; progression; and breathing should produce excellent results.

Range of Motion and Speed Each repetition should take 4 to 6 seconds: 2 to 3 seconds for the lifting movement and 2 to 3 seconds for the lowering movement. Controlling the lowering phase emphasizes the stronger negative muscle contraction and should increase the productivity of each exercise set. It is also important to perform each repetition through a full range of motion. This enhances both joint integrity and flexibility.

Loads, Repetitions, and Sets The recommended exercises in tables 11.13 to 11.15 are listed from the larger muscles of the legs to the smaller muscles of the neck and should be performed in this order. One or two sets of each exercise are sufficient, as long as you train using good form to the point of muscle fatigue. Because intensity is the key to strength development, use enough resistance to fatigue the target muscle groups in about 30 to 90 seconds. In general, this is achieved with a weight load that you can lift for 8 to 12 controlled repetitions at 4 to 6 seconds each.

Frequency If you play tennis three or four days per week, it is probably best to strength train on two nontennis days. If you practice tennis every day, perform resistance exercise about four hours after your tennis training for best overall results. For example, if you play tennis every morning from 9:00 to 11:00, schedule your strength exercise around 3:00 p.m. Strength training once a week or on two days spaced evenly through the week is sufficient for building strength that will improve your tennis game.

Progression As your muscles become stronger, it is essential to progressively increase the work effort. This is best accomplished by gradually increasing the exercise resistance. Once you complete 12 repetitions, the weight load is no longer heavy enough to produce maximum strength benefits. By increasing the resistance about 5 percent (typically 1 to 5 pounds [.45 to 2.5 kg]), you can continue to stimulate strength development.

Breathing It is essential to breathe on every repetition because holding your breath can lead to undesirable increases in blood pressure and restricted blood flow. Exhale during each lifting movement and inhale during each lowering movement.

Strength Exercises for Tennis Players

Tennis players can improve strength and endurance by performing a variety of exercises using machines, free weights, or body-weight and resistance band training. Tables 11.13 to 11.15 present our recommended strength training exercises for tennis players, which provide a solid conditioning base for improved tennis performance, and the order in which they should be performed in the workout. These exercises should also reduce your risk of injury, especially when complemented by exercises for the shoulder rotator cuff and forearm discussed earlier.

Table 11.13 Strength Training for Tennis Players: Machine Exercises

Exercise	Muscle group	Page #
1. Leg press	Quadriceps, hamstrings, gluteals	62
2. Hip abduction	Hip adductors	65
3. Hip adduction	Hip abductors	64
4. Heel raise	Gastrocnemius, soleus	66
5. Chest press	Pectoralis major, anterior deltoids, triceps	71
6. Seated row	Latissimus dorsi, teres major, rhomboids, middle trapezius, biceps, posterior deltoids	79
7. Shoulder press	Deltoids, upper trapezius, triceps	74
8. Biceps curl	Biceps	84
9. Triceps extension	Triceps	85
10. Abdominal flexion	Core: Rectus abdominis	68
11. Low back extension	Core: Erector spinae	67
12. Rotary torso	Core: Rectus abdominis, internal obliques, external obliques	69
13. Neck flexion and extension	Neck flexors, neck extensors	89, 88

Training load	Repetitions	Sets	Repetition speed	Recovery time
70-80% max	8-12	1-2	4-6 sec	60-90 sec

Table 11.14 Strength Training for Tennis Players: Free-Weight Exercises

Exercise	Muscle group	Page #
1. Barbell or dumbbell squat	Quadriceps, hamstrings, gluteals	94, 92
2. Dumbbell lunge	Quadriceps, hamstrings, gluteals	97
3. Barbell, dumbbell, or kettlebell heel raise	Gastrocnemius, soleus	100, 98
4. Barbell or dumbbell bench press	Pectoralis major, anterior deltoids, triceps	112, 110
5. Dumbbell double bent-over row	Latissimus dorsi, teres minor, rhomboids, middle trapezius, biceps, posterior deltoids	128
6. Dumbbell alternating shoulder press	Deltoids, upper trapezius, triceps	120
7. Dumbbell pullover	Latissimus dorsi, teres major, triceps	124
8. Body-weight trunk curl*	Core: Rectus abdominis	154
9. Body-weight trunk extension*	Core: Erector spinae	150
10. Body-weight twisting trunk curl*	Core: Rectus abdominis, internal obliques, external obliques, hip flexors, rectus femoris	152
11. Barbell or dumbbell shrug	Upper trapezius	140, 141
12. Wrist roller	Forearm flexors, forearm extensors	230

Training load	Repetitions	Sets	Repetition speed	Recovery time
70-80% max	8-12	1-2	4-6 sec	60-90 sec

*Body-weight exercises: As many repetitions as necessary to fatigue the target muscles.

Table 11.15 Strength Training for Tennis Players: Body-Weight and Resistance Band Exercises

Exercise	Muscle group	Page #
1. Wall squat: exercise ball*	Quadriceps, hamstrings, gluteals	144
2. Exercise ball heel pull*	Hamstrings, hip flexors	145
3. Exercise ball leg lift*	Quadriceps, hip flexors, rectus abdominis	146
4. Body-weight push-up*	Pectoralis major, anterior deltoids, triceps, rectus abdominis	160
5. Resistance band seated row	Latissimus dorsi, teres major, rhomboids, middle trapezius, biceps, posterior deltoids	168
6. Resistance band seated press	Deltoids, upper trapezius, triceps	164
7. Body-weight bench dip*	Pectoralis major, anterior deltoids, triceps	171
8. Body-weight trunk curl*	Core: Rectus abdominis	154
9. Body-weight trunk extension*	Core: Erector spinae	150
10. Body-weight twisting trunk curl*	Core: Rectus abdominis, internal obliques, external obliques	152
11. Resistance band shrug	Upper trapezius	175

Training load	Repetitions	Sets	Repetition speed	Recovery time
70-80% max	8-12	1-2	4-6 sec	60-90 sec

*Body-weight exercises: As many repetitions as necessary to fatigue the target muscles.

Summary for Tennis

Remember that skill training is the most important factor in improving your tennis game. However, physical conditioning can certainly enhance your playing efforts and outcomes. The cornerstone of physical conditioning is muscular strength, and a stronger tennis player should always be a better tennis player. Be sure to eat enough calories to fuel your combined physical activities, including more protein and lots of water. Finally, try to sleep at least eight hours nightly so that you enter every exercise session with energy and enthusiasm.

Exercise selection	Include appropriate exercises to cumulatively address all of the major muscle groups.
Training load	Use a training load that is 70 to 80 percent of maximum resistance.
Repetitions	Complete 8 to 12 controlled repetitions.
Progression	Increase the resistance by 5 percent when you can complete 12 repetitions in 2 successive sessions.
Sets	Complete 1 or 2 sets of each exercise.
Movement speed	Complete each movement at a moderate speed, taking 2 to 3 seconds to lift and 2 to 3 seconds to lower.
Movement range	Perform each movement through a relatively full range of motion.
Training frequency	Complete 1 or 2 exercise sessions per week.

STRENGTH TRAINING FOR GOLFERS

You, like more than 50 million Americans, enjoy playing golf. If you are like most golfers, you want to play more golf, at a higher level, with no injuries. We refer to this as playing stronger and driving longer, both of which can be accomplished through a well-designed strength training program.

Our approach to golf conditioning involves two brief exercise sessions a week, leaving plenty of time for practicing and playing your sport. Each workout includes strength training, stretching exercises, and optional aerobic activity. Golfers have traditionally avoided strength training for fear of adding body weight, developing large muscles, feeling tight, losing speed, compromising coordination, developing errant drives, and posting higher scores. However, our research has shown significant benefits to golfers who perform regular strength training (Westcott, Dolan, and Cavicchi 1996). As you can see in table 11.16, the 77 adult golfers who completed just two months of our strength training program made impressive improvements in their health, fitness, and driving power (Draovitch and Westcott 1999). Golfers who followed our program reduced their resting blood pressure by almost 5 mmHg, increased their strength by more than 50 percent, lost 4 pounds (1.8 kg) of fat, added 4 pounds (1.8 kg) of muscle, and increased their club-head speed (driving power) by 6 percent.

Our golf conditioning participants attained greater increases in club-head speed when they combined stretching exercise with the strength training program (Westcott and Parziale 1997). They performed six basic stretches for the major muscle groups, including the thighs, hips, lower back, upper back, chest, and shoulders. They performed each stretch slowly, with a 20-second stationary hold in the fully stretched position. If you have time, stretch after each strength training session to develop the flexibility that will contribute to improved club-head speed.

In simple terms, power is muscular force multiplied by movement distance divided by movement time. You may recall reading about this in the first part of this chapter. You can improve your driving power by increasing your muscle force, increasing your swing distance, decreasing your swing time, or a combination of any of these. Strength training is the best means for increasing your muscular force, and including stretching exercises is the best means for increasing your swing distance. Decreasing your swing time is a more complex task involving practice and coordination; however, stronger muscles and more flexible joints will also help you increase the speed of your swing.

Table 11.16 Results of Eight-Week Strength Training Program for Golfers

	Change	Amount
Mean resting blood pressure	Decrease	4.5 mm Hg
Muscle	Increase	56%
Body weight	Decrease	.2 lb (.9 kg)
Percent fat	Decrease	2%
Fat weight	Decrease	4.1 lb (1.9 kg)
Muscle weight	Increase	3.9 lb (1.8 kg)
Club-head speed	Increase	6.1%

$$Power = muscular\ force\ \times\ \frac{movement\ distance}{movement\ time}$$

Although we did not measure cardiorespiratory conditioning in our research studies on golf, we asked the golfers in the program to choose their favorite endurance exercise (walking, jogging, cycling, stepping) or a combination of these to promote a cross-training effect. We encourage you to include regular aerobic activity in your golf training program. This aerobic activity takes 20 to 30 minutes, including a few minutes for warming up and cooling down, and occurs on three nonconsecutive days each week. Using an effort scale of 1 to 10, perform the warm-up and cool-down segments at a low intensity (levels 3 to 4) and the conditioning segment at a moderate intensity (levels 6 to 7). Although improved cardiorespiratory fitness has little direct impact on your driving power, it may enable you to play stronger and longer by increasing your resistance to fatigue and your ability to concentrate.

Program Design for Golfers

The exercises in the strength training program for golfers do not imitate specific movements or emphasize specific muscles; rather, they focus on the exercises that strengthen all of the muscle groups used in golf. The following guidelines for range of motion and speed; loads, repetitions, and sets; frequency; progression; and breathing should produce excellent results.

Range of Motion and Speed   Perform each repetition at a moderate speed of 4 to 6 seconds, taking 2 to 3 seconds to lift the resistance and 2 to 3 seconds to lower it. Perform each repetition through a full range of motion if you can do so without discomfort.

Loads, Repetitions, and Sets   Train with a load that enables you to complete 8 to 12 repetitions to the point of momentary fatigue. This is 70 to 80 percent of your maximum resistance, which is a productive training load for increasing strength. Perform 1 or 2 sets of each of the training exercises presented in tables 11.17 to 11.19.

Frequency   Although one weekly workout is sufficient, you will improve your physical fitness and increase your driving power more quickly by training on two or three nonconsecutive days each week. However, if your time is limited, one session a week will produce results, preferably on a nongolfing day.

Progression   When you can complete 12 repetitions using correct technique during two successive workouts, increase the training load by approximately 5 percent (typically 1 to 5 pounds [.45 to 2.5 kg]).

Breathing   Breathe during each repetition because holding your breath can lead to undesirable increases in blood pressure and restricted blood flow. Exhale during each lifting movement and inhale during each lowering movement.

Strength Exercises for Golfers

The following sections present the recommended exercises, training principles, and workout progressions for improving your muscular strength. Let's begin with the muscles of the trunk. They are important for two reasons. First, many golfers have problems in the low back caused largely by weak trunk muscles, particularly the erector spinae muscles in the low back. Second, the trunk muscles play a key role in transferring the power produced by the large hip and thigh muscles to the club-swinging muscles of the upper body and arms.

The second group of muscles golfers should strengthen are those of the thighs and hips. The muscles at the front of the thigh (quadriceps) and rear of the thigh (hamstrings) are major generators of force, especially in conjunction with the gluteal muscles of the hips. The leg press and squat exercises are ideal for strengthening these large muscle groups. Because weight transfer and hip thrust are critical components of powerful golf drives, we also recommend specific strength exercises for the inner-thigh muscles (hip adductors) and outer-thigh muscles (hip abductors).

The third group of muscles that contributes to driving power includes the chest muscles (pectoralis major), upper-back muscles (latissimus dorsi), and shoulder muscles (deltoids). These muscles produce the swinging action of the arms and also control shoulder joint movements. It is, therefore, important to maintain balanced strength in these muscles in order to reduce the risk of shoulder joint injuries. Because making contact with the ball requires that you keep your head stable, we also recommended exercises that strengthen the neck.

Golfers can increase strength, endurance, and power by performing a variety of exercises using machines, free weights, or body-weight and resistance band training. Tables 11.17 to 11.19 present our recommended strength training exercise for golfers and the order in which they should be performed in the workout.

Table 11.17   Strength Training for Golfers: Machine Exercises

Exercise	Muscle group	Page #
1. Leg press	Quadriceps, hamstrings, gluteals	62
2. Hip abduction	Hip abductors	65
3. Hip adduction	Hip adductors	64
4. Heel raise	Gastrocnemius, soleus	66
5. Chest crossover	Pectoralis major, anterior deltoids, serratus anterior	70
6. Pullover	Latissimus dorsi, teres major, triceps	76
7. Lateral raise	Deltoids	73
8. Biceps curl	Biceps	84
9. Triceps extension	Triceps	85
10. Abdominal flexion	Core: Rectus abdominis	68
11. Low back extension	Core: Erector spinae	67
12. Rotary torso	Core: Rectus abdominis, internal obliques, external obliques	69
13. Neck flexion and extension	Neck flexors, neck extensors	89, 88

Training load	Repetitions	Sets	Repetition speed	Recovery time
70-80% max	8-12	1-2	4-6 sec	60-90 sec

Table 11.18   Strength Training for Golfers: Free-Weight Exercises

Exercise	Muscle group	Page #
1. Barbell or dumbbell squat	Quadriceps, hamstrings, gluteals	94, 92
2. Barbell or dumbbell lunge	Quadriceps, hamstrings, gluteals	97
3. Barbell, dumbbell, or kettlebell heel raise	Gastrocnemius, soleus	100, 98
4. Dumbbell chest fly	Pectoralis major, anterior deltoids, serratus anterior	109
5. Dumbbell pullover	Latissimus dorsi, teres major, triceps	124
6. Dumbbell lateral raise	Deltoids	118
7. Dumbbell curl	Biceps	130
8. Dumbbell overhead triceps extension	Triceps	135
9. Body-weight trunk curl*	Core: Rectus abdominis	154
10. Body-weight trunk extension*	Core: Erector spinae	150
11. Body-weight twisting trunk curl*	Core: Rectus abdominis, internal obliques, external obliques, hip flexors, rectus femoris	152
12. Barbell or dumbbell shrug	Upper trapezius	140, 141
13. Wrist roller	Forearm flexors, forearm extensors	230

Training load	Repetitions	Sets	Repetition speed	Recovery time
70-80% max	8-12	1-2	4-6 sec	60-90 sec

*Body-weight exercises: As many repetitions as necessary to fatigue the target muscles.

Table 11.19   Strength Training for Golfers: Body-Weight and Resistance Band Exercises

Exercise	Muscle group	Page #
1. Wall squat: exercise ball*	Quadriceps, hamstrings, gluteals	144
2. Exercise ball heel pull*	Hamstrings, hip flexors	145
3. Exercise ball leg lift*	Quadriceps, hip flexors, rectus abdominis	146
4. Resistance band chest press	Pectoralis major, anterior deltoids, triceps	159
5. Resistance band seated row	Latissimus dorsi, teres major, rhomboids, middle trapezius, biceps, posterior deltoids	168
6. Resistance band seated press	Deltoids, upper trapezius, triceps	164
7. Body-weight push-up*	Pectoralis major, anterior deltoids, triceps, rectus abdominis	160
8. Body-weight trunk curl*	Core: Rectus abdominis	154
9. Body-weight trunk extension*	Core: Erector spinae	150
10. Body-weight twisting trunk curl*	Core: Rectus abdominis, internal obliques, external obliques, hip flexors, rectus femoris	152
11. Resistance band shrug	Upper trapezius	175

Training load	Repetitions	Sets	Repetition speed	Recovery time
70-80% max	8-12	1-2	4-6 sec	60-90 sec

*Body-weight exercises: As many repetitions as necessary to fatigue the target muscles.

Summary for Golf Conditioning

Keep accurate records of your workouts, and watch how your driving power correlates to your strength development. Be sure to eat enough calories to fuel your combined physical activities, including more protein and lots of water. Finally, try to sleep at least eight hours nightly so that you enter every exercise session with energy and enthusiasm.

Exercise selection	Include appropriate exercises to cumulatively address all of the major muscle groups.
Training load	Use a training load that is approximately 70 to 80 percent of maximum resistance.
Repetitions	Complete 8 to 12 controlled repetitions.
Progression	Increase the resistance by 5 percent when you can lift 12 repetitions in 2 successive sessions.
Sets	Complete 1 or 2 sets of each exercise.
Movement speed	Complete each movement at a moderate speed, taking 2 to 3 seconds to lift and 2 to 3 seconds to lower.
Movement range	Perform each exercise through a relatively full range of motion.
Training frequency	Complete at least 1, but preferably 2 or 3, exercise sessions per week.

12

Nutrition for Continual Improvement

Your dietary habits have a major impact on your body weight, body composition, and physical health. Unfortunately, most Americans consume too many calories for the amount of activity they perform. As a result, about three out of four older adults in the United States are overweight, which predisposes them to increased risk of diabetes, heart disease, joint problems, and many types of cancer (Flegal et al. 2010; Westcott 2012). At the same time, consuming too little protein, calcium, or vitamin D can cause a weakening of the musculoskeletal system and lead to osteoporosis; insufficient iron in your diet may cause you to become anemic; and excessive sodium intake may contribute to hypertension.

Eating foods high in fiber, low in trans fat, and rich in vitamins and minerals is essential for optimal health and disease prevention. For example, vitamins A and C, found in many fruits and vegetables, are considered important antioxidants (nutritional bodyguards) that protect against potentially harmful chemical reactions in body cells. Potassium, found in bananas, cantaloupe, and avocados, is involved in every muscle contraction and, therefore, is especially important for people participating in strength training.

Although you can consume vitamins and minerals through nutritional supplements, do not be tempted to substitute supplements for a balanced diet that includes a variety of vegetables, fruits, and whole grains as well as lean meats and low-fat dairy products. Human nutrient requirements are too complex (and too poorly understood) to be adequately accommodated by pills, and only a varied (well-rounded) diet can provide the proper foundation for optimal nutrition. We recommend following the guidelines for daily food choices set forth by the United States Department of Agriculture in the MyPlate Plan (see figure 12.1).

Keep in mind that a balanced diet is not the same as a low-calorie diet designed for losing weight. Reduced-calorie diets should be approved by

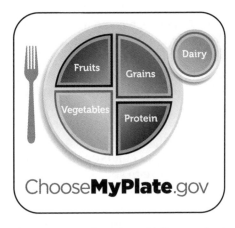

Figure 12.1 Follow the guidelines set forth by the USDA in the MyPlate plan.

USDA Center for Nutrition Policy and Promotion

your physician or a registered dietitian, especially when you are following the strength training programs presented in this text.

PROTEIN INTAKE FOR PEOPLE PAST 50

The strength training programs presented in chapters 9, 10, and 11 produce various levels of muscle microtrauma that stimulate tissue-building processes for developing larger and stronger muscles. Of course, the physiological mechanisms for muscle synthesis require sufficient supplies of the amino acid building blocks contained in protein-rich foods.

We advocate a sensible nutrition plan for people past age 50, similar in most respects to that recommended for younger adults. However, during the past few years it has become clear that older adults should increase their protein consumption as they age. Dr. Wayne Campbell, one of the leading nutrition researchers in the United States, has stated that people over age 50 who eat the recommended daily allowance (RDA) of protein (approximately 0.4 g protein per pound of body weight or 0.8 g protein per kg of body weight) will lose muscle mass even if they participate regularly in strength training (Campbell et al. 2001; Schardt 2007). Dr. Campbell's research indicates that people over age 50 who perform resistance exercise need at least 25 percent more protein than the RDA (approximately 0.5 g protein per pound of body weight or 1.0 g protein per kg of body weight) to maintain muscle mass and at least 50 percent more protein than the RDA (approximately 0.6 g protein per pound of body weight or 1.2 g protein per kg of body weight) to increase muscle mass.

This is the case primarily because older adults do not assimilate protein (amino acids) nearly as well as they did earlier in life. Research conducted at the University of Texas revealed that the older participants (average age 68 years) assimilated 61 percent fewer amino acids from protein sources consumed compared to the younger participants (average age 31 years) (Katsanos et al. 2005). Because amino acids are the building blocks for muscle tissue, these research results have important implications for all who want to attain and maintain muscular fitness.

In 2013 we published a study on protein consumption in the medical research journal *Physician and Sportsmedicine*. The strength training participants who increased their protein intake to 0.7 gram per pound of body weight (1.5 g per kg of body weight) gained significantly more lean (muscle) weight than the strength training participants who maintained their normal protein intake. Based on our findings, we recommend that men and women over age 50 consume 0.6 to 0.7 gram of protein per pound of body weight to maximize the effects of strength training programs.

According to numerous research studies, the best time to consume additional protein is close to your strength training session. In another study on protein and resistance exercise (Westcott et al. 2011), the participants who consumed a protein shake at the conclusion of their weight workout had greater increases in both muscle mass and bone density than those who did not drink the protein shake. Our study and many others with similar results provided the participants with approximately 25 grams of protein shortly after they finished training.

Taking into consideration the greater protein intake requirements for older adults, we recommend that strength exercisers ages 50 to 80 may benefit from 50 to 70 percent more daily protein than the minimum levels recommended in the RDA guidelines.

Table 12.1 presents the recommended allowance for daily protein intake for men and women over age 50 along with our guidelines on daily protein consumption for those in their 50s, 60s, and 70s who perform regular strength training. Table 12.2 lists the grams of protein found in a variety of protein-rich foods. It also lists standard portion sizes.

In addition to consuming sufficient protein for tissue building and muscle development, senior strength trainers should pay close attention to the distribution of their protein ingestion. Rather than eating all of your protein-rich foods at one meal, it is better to distribute your protein intake throughout the day to enhance amino acid assimilation. For example, snacks such as a glass of milk, a yogurt smoothie, a protein shake, a hard-boiled egg, or half a sandwich made with tuna, turkey, or peanut butter provide excellent sources of protein. Also be sure to consume extra protein soon after completing your strength training workouts.

Table 12.1 Adjusted Minimum Daily Protein Recommendations

Age ranges in years	Recommended daily protein intake	Percent increase for strength trainers	Recommended daily protein intake for strength trainers
50-59	Men: 56 grams	Men: 50%	Men: 85 grams
	Women: 46 grams	Women: 50%	Women: 70 grams
60-69	Men: 56 grams	Men: 60%	Men: 90 grams
	Women: 46 grams	Women: 60%	Women: 75 grams
70-79	Men: 56 grams	Men: 70%	Men: 95 grams
	Women: 46 grams	Women: 70%	Women: 80 grams

Table 12.2 Grams of Protein in Protein-Rich Foods

Food	Portion size	Protein grams per serving
Tuna	6 oz (175 g)	45
Chicken (white meat)	6 oz (175 g)	45
Protein powder	6 tbsp in 8 oz (250 ml) of milk	36
Yogurt smoothie	20 oz (600ml)	20
Greek yogurt (plain)	8 oz (250 ml)	20
Milk (low fat)	16 oz (500 ml)	16
Peanut butter	4 tbsp	14
Eggs	2	12

Certainly, protein is a key nutrient for optimal development of your musculoskeletal system. However, it is essential to design a well-balanced nutrition plan that includes all of the basic nutrients in appropriate amounts for overall physiological function and performance power. Read and apply the nutrition information in the following sections to maximize the effectiveness of your strength training program. When it comes to food, it is always best to begin with the basics.

BASIC NUTRIENTS

As shown in figure 12.1, the MyPlate Plan is high in carbohydrate, moderate in protein, and low in fat. The carbohydrate choices are divided into grains, vegetables, and fruits. The suggested protein sources are dairy products and lean meats, and the recommended fat-rich foods are vegetable oils used sparingly. Approximately half of your food intake should be from fruits and vegetables and the remainder derived somewhat evenly from lean meats, dairy products, and grains. Let's consider each of the food categories more carefully.

Grains

Grains include all kinds of foods made from wheat, oats, corn, rice, and the like. Examples of grain foods are cereals, breads, pasta, pancakes, rice cakes, tortillas, bagels, muffins, cornbread, rice pudding, and chocolate cake. Potatoes, because of their high carbohydrate content, are also included in the grains category. Obviously, some grain-based foods, such as cakes, cookies, and pastries, contain a lot of sugar and trans fat, so you should eat them sparingly.

All grains are high in carbohydrate, and some grains or parts of grains, such as wheat germ, are also good sources of protein. Whole grains are typically rich in B vitamins and fiber. Grains are plentiful and inexpensive and should be part of every meal. MyPlate recommends that approximately one-quarter of your daily food intake come from grains and that at least half of your grain foods be whole grams. A serving of grain is equivalent to a slice of bread or a half cup of cooked pasta, so if you consume 6 ounces (180 g) of grains a day, 3 ounces (90 g) should be from whole-grain sources. Consider using brown rice, whole-wheat pasta, and whole-grain cereals to attain more whole grains in your diet. Refer to the box for sample exchange units for popular food choices in the grains category.

Vegetables

Like grains, vegetables are excellent sources of carbohydrate, vitamins, and fiber. Vegetables come in all sizes, shapes, colors, and nutritional characteristics, and they are relatively low in calories. Orange vegetables are typically good sources of vitamin A and beta-carotene. This category includes carrots and winter squash.

Green vegetables are characteristically high in vitamin B_2 and folic acid. Some of the many green vegetables are peas, beans, broccoli, asparagus, spinach, and lettuce. Red vegetables generally provide ample amounts of vitamin C. The best known vegetables in this category are tomatoes and red peppers. Other vegetables

Sample Exchange Units Equivalent to One Serving of Grain

Cereals

¼ cup nugget cereal (Grape-Nuts)

⅓ cup concentrated bran cereal

½ cup cooked hot cereal (oatmeal or Cream of Wheat)

¾ cup flaked cereal

1 ½ cups puffed cereal

Breads

½ bagel or English muffin

1 slice bread

1 piece of pita bread

1 tortilla

Grains

¼ cup wheat germ

⅓ cup brown or white rice

½ cup pasta, macaroni, or noodles

½ cup hominy, barley, or grits

Snacks

¾ oz (22.5 g) pretzels

¾ oz (22.5 g) rice cakes

4 crackers (1 oz, or 30 g)

3 cups air-popped popcorn

Note: 1 cup (imperial) = .946 cup (metric) = 1.041 cup (Canada).

are essentially white, at least under the skin. These include cauliflower, summer squash, and radishes, many of which are good sources of vitamin C.

The MyPlate Plan recommends that approximately a quarter of your daily food intake be vegetables. One serving is half a cup of any raw vegetable, except for lettuce and sprouts, which require one cup per serving. Because heating reduces water content, cooked vegetables require less space than uncooked vegetables and serving sizes may be smaller. Likewise, vegetable juices are more concentrated and require only half a cup per serving. MyPlate suggests that you choose vegetables that are rich in color, especially red, orange, and dark green.

It is a good idea to eat some of your vegetables raw and to steam or microwave other vegetables for nutrient retention. In addition, fresh or frozen vegetables have more nutritional value and are lower in sodium than canned vegetables.

Fruit

Fruits are the counterpart to vegetables: relatively low in calories, with as much variety and nutritional value. Essentially all fruit choices are high in carbohydrate and vitamins, and many provide excellent sources of fiber.

Citrus fruits, such as oranges, grapefruit, and lemons, are loaded with vitamin C. Like orange-colored vegetables, orange-colored fruits, including cantaloupe, apricots, and papaya, are rich in vitamin A and beta-carotene. Both green fruits, such as honeydew melon and kiwi, and red fruits, such as strawberries and cherries, are high in vitamin C.

Yellow fruits include peaches, mangos, and pineapples, all of which are good sources of vitamin C. Fruits that are white, at least on the inside, include apples, pears, and bananas, all of which are high in potassium. Avocadoes are also rich sources of potassium and contain much fiber and healthy fat.

Dried fruits are particularly nutrient dense. Raisins, dates, figs, and prunes are all superb energy sources, and prunes are the best source of dietary fiber.

The MyPlate Plan recommends that, like vegetables, fruit intake be approximately one-quarter of your daily food consumption. The box presents sample exchange quantities for a variety of fruits. You will notice that one serving varies considerably, depending on the type of fruit you eat. For example, it takes a quarter of a melon or half of a grapefruit to equal three dates or two tablespoons of raisins. The difference is water content. Fresh fruits contain lots of water, whereas dried fruits are essentially high-density carbohydrate. If you prefer your fruits in liquid form, half a cup (125 ml) of fruit juice equals one serving but has less fiber than whole fruit. MyPlate suggests that you eat fruit at breakfast, lunch, and dinner as well as use dried fruits for snacks.

Sample Exchange Units
Equivalent to One Serving of Fruit

2 tbsp (18 g) raisins	¾ cup pineapple
3 dates	2 kiwi
3 prunes	½ pomegranate
½ cup grapes	¼ cantaloupe
¾ cup berries	¼ papaya
1 apple	¼ melon
1 banana	½ mango
1 peach	5 kumquat
1 pear	1 cup honeydew
3 apricots	1¼ cups strawberries
½ grapefruit	1¼ cups watermelon

Dairy Products

The MyPlate plan recommends daily dairy consumption in addition to other protein sources. Low-fat dairy products are preferred, which include milk, yogurt, and cheese. These foods are excellent sources of protein and calcium. Because whole-milk products are high in fat and therefore calories, you should be selective in the dairy section. For example, 1 percent milk, low-fat yogurt, and nonfat cottage cheese offer heart-healthy alternatives to higher-fat dairy selections.

Refer to the Sample Exchange Units Equivalent to One Serving of Dairy box for exchange units equivalent to one serving of dairy. Notice that a quarter cup of low-fat cottage cheese and 1 cup (250 ml) of 1 percent milk have similar nutritional values. Although there are many sources of dietary protein, you may have difficulty obtaining sufficient calcium unless you regularly consume milk products. If you have problems digesting milk, try to regularly consume other foods that are high in calcium, such as tofu, leafy greens, beans, broccoli, and sesame seeds. MyPlate suggests trying lactose-free milk, soy milk, or smaller amounts of milk at a time.

Sample Exchange Units Equivalent to One Serving of Dairy

1 oz (30 g) cheese	½ cup evaporated milk
¼ cup cottage cheese	1 cup milk
¼ cup ricotta cheese	1 cup yogurt
¼ cup Parmesan cheese	1 cup buttermilk

Protein Foods

According to the MyPlate plan, this category includes meat, poultry, seafood, eggs, beans, peas, soy products, nuts, and seeds. All these foods are good sources of protein, although some also contain significant amounts of fat. Table 12.3 lists foods in the protein category according to their fat content. Note that how meat is prepared often affects its fat content. We'll look at this aspect in more detail in the food preparation section.

Although there are differences in fat content, protein exchange units are consistent among the foods in this category. As you can see from the Sample Exchange Units Equivalent to One Serving of Protein box, 3 ounces (90 g) of meat, poultry, and fish (about the size of a deck of cards) have equal exchange values, as do a half cup of dry beans and a half cup of tuna. MyPlate recommends that approximately one-quarter of your daily food intake be from protein sources. Refer to the box for sample exchange units for popular food choices in the protein category.

Table 12.3 Foods in Meat and Bean Group Categorized by Fat Content

Low fat	Medium fat	High fat
Most fish	Chicken with skin	Beef ribs
Egg whites	Turkey with skin	Pork ribs
Chicken without skin	Roast beef	Corned beef
Turkey without skin	Roast pork	Sausage
Venison	Roast lamb	Lunch meat
Rabbit	Veal cutlet	Ground pork
Top round	Ground beef	Hot dogs
Eye of round	Steaks	Fried chicken
Sirloin tenderloin	Canned salmon	Fried fish
Flank steak	Oil-packed tuna	Nuts*
Veal	Whole eggs	Peanuts*
Dry beans	Pork chops	Peanut butter*

* Note that these foods, although high in fat, are quite healthy and are shown to aid in raising HDL (good) cholesterol and lowering LDL (bad) cholesterol.

Sample Exchange Units
Equivalent to One Serving of Protein

3 oz (90 g) fish

3 oz (90 g) poultry

3 oz (90 g) meat (e.g., beef, poultry, lamb)

1 egg or 2 egg whites

4 tbsp peanut butter

½ cup cooked dry beans

½ cup tuna

½ cup tofu

6 tbsp (53 g) nuts

Sodium, Solid Fat, Added Sugar, and Oil

MyPlate recommends cutting down on foods containing high amounts of sodium, solid fat, and added sugar. It is also advisable to limit consumption of oils because oils and fat contain 9 calories per gram. Use the box to determine serving equivalents for foods in the fat group. Trans fat (such as found in many commercially baked goods) poses a significant health risk; therefore, avoid this type of fat as much as possible.

Sample Exchange Units
Equivalent to One Serving of Fat

1 tsp butter	1 tbsp diet mayonnaise
1 tsp margarine	1 tsp oil
1 tbsp diet margarine	1 tbsp salad dressing
1 tsp mayonnaise	

Note: 1 U.S. tsp = 5 ml; 1 U.S. tbsp = 15 ml.

2 tbsp diet salad dressing	2 tbsp sour cream
1 tbsp cream cheese	4 tbsp light sour cream
2 tbsp light cream cheese	2 tbsp coffee creamer (liquid)

Water

Water is not included in the MyPlate Plan because it contains no calories and is not technically a food. Nonetheless, it is the most important nutrient for your body. Your body is mostly water (even your muscles are about 75 percent water), and you can live only a few days without taking in water.

The standard recommendation is to drink six to eight 8-ounce (250 ml) glasses of water daily, and even more water is desirable when you exercise. Unfortunately, natural thirst mechanism declines with age, so active adults should monitor water consumption to ensure they drink 6 to 8 glasses every day. It is advisable to drink a glass of water before and after each strength training session as well as throughout your workout. Remember that muscle tissue is more than three-quarters water.

Because coffee, tea, diet drinks, and alcoholic beverages have a diuretic effect, they are not as effective for hydration as seltzer and fruit juices. Apple juice is an excellent source of potassium, and, of course, orange juice is high in vitamin C. Cranberry juice is close to orange juice in vitamin C content and may help prevent bladder infections. Carrot juice is high in vitamin A, vitamin C, potassium, and fiber. Pomegranate juice is reported to be the highest in antioxidants. Low-fat milk is mostly water and an excellent source of protein, calcium, and vitamin D. Sport drinks are also acceptable substitutes for water, but like fruit juices and low-fat milk, they are high in calories.

THREE STEPS TO BETTER NUTRITION

An eating program that provides all essential nutrients requires careful food selection, substitution, and preparation. The following suggestions should help you implement your best dietary intentions.

Food Selection

If you use the MyPlate Plan guidelines for grains, vegetables, fruits, dairy products, and protein, your diet will be generally high in nutrition. The following foods contain less saturated fat than other choices in their category.:

- Fish
- Poultry without skin
- Low-fat milk, yogurt, cottage cheese
- Olive, peanut, sunflower, safflower, corn, and canola oils

Note: Avoid prepared foods that contain trans fat, which is listed on container labels as partially hydrogenated vegetable oil.

Food Substitution

You undoubtedly have certain favorite foods that you do not want to give up. You may be surprised to discover that simple substitutions can reduce the fat content without detracting from the taste. For example, using evaporated skim milk in place of cream cuts the calorie content by more than 65 percent. Another practical substitution is to use plain nonfat yogurt or nonfat sour cream in place of standard sour cream on baked potatoes. Doing so reduces the calorie content and supplies your body with twice as much beneficial calcium.

Other substitutes are herbs rather than table salt, low-fat frozen yogurt instead of ice cream, cocoa powder in place of chocolate squares in baked goods, and lemon juice or vinegar with olive oil instead of bottled salad dressings.

If you have a sweet tooth, try eating fresh fruit in place of candy, cookies, and baked goods. If you prefer crunchy snacks like potato chips, you may appreciate lower-calorie alternatives such as pretzels (watch the sodium, though), baked chips, or carrot sticks. Nuts contain heart-healthy fat, vitamins, and protein; therefore, they are a good substitute for chips and sweets.

Food Preparation

How you prepare your food may increase or decrease the healthfulness. For example, frying can double and triple the calories in some foods. By using a nonfat vegetable spray or a nonstick skillet, you can eliminate the oils typically necessary for frying. Baked or broiled meats are recommended, and steamed or microwaved vegetables are suggested for nutrient retention. Avoid adding butter and salt to vegetables during the cooking process. If you prefer, apply these sparingly to suit individual taste once the servings are on your plate. This is because it takes less salt and fat to enhance the taste of food after cooking than during cooking.

SAMPLE DAILY MENU PLANS

Tables 12.4 through 12.6 present three sample daily menu plans based on the MyPlate recommendations for balanced meals and healthy eating. These sample menu plans provide approximately 2,000 calories daily. The MyPlate recommended servings for the five food categories (grains, vegetables, fruits, dairy, and protein) are as follows for a 2,000-calorie-per-day nutrition plan.

Grains	Approximately 6 ounces a day (preferably whole grains).
Vegetables	Approximately 2.5 cups a day (preferably colorful vegetables).
Fruits	Approximately 2 cups a day (including fruit juices and dried fruits).
Dairy	Approximately 3 cups a day (preferably low-fat milk, yogurt, and cheese options).
Protein foods	Approximately 5.5 ounces a day (preferably fish, chicken, turkey, and lean meats).

You will note that the sample menu plans may include a midmorning, midafternoon, and midevening snack in addition to three balanced meals of breakfast, lunch, and dinner. Although these are typically minimeals, many of the suggested snacks provide extra protein that appears to be beneficial for optimal muscle development. Of course, the sample menu plans are merely models that may be modified as you desire. Just try to maintain an appropriate daily caloric intake and a balanced nutrient intake consistent with the protein guidelines presented earlier in this chapter.

Table 12.4 Menu 1

Food	Portion/calories
Breakfast	
Waffles	2/174
Butter	1 tbsp/102
Peanut butter	2 tbsp/188
Banana	1 small/93
Skim milk	8 oz (250 ml)/86
Snack	
Wheat crackers	16/160
Lunch	
Tuna	3 oz (90 g)/110
Mayonnaise	1 tbsp/100
Wheat bread	2 slices/130
Lettuce and tomato	1/2 cup/10
Skim milk	8 oz (250 ml)/86
Apple	1/80
Snack	
Pear	1/100
Dinner	
Skim milk	8 oz (250 ml)/86
Pasta	1 cup/197
Tomato sauce	1/2 cup/71
Zucchini	1/2 cup/14
Ground turkey	2 oz (60 g)/84
Garlic bread	1 slice/82
with butter	1 tbsp/102
Snack	
Celery sticks	1/2 cup/10

Table 12.5 Menu 2

Food	Portion/calories
Breakfast	
Orange juice	6 oz (175 ml)/86
Honey Bunches of Oats cereal	2 oz (60 g)/223
Skim milk	8 oz (250 ml)/86
Lunch	
Turkey	3 oz (90 g)/161
Swiss cheese	1 oz (30 g)/95
Tomato	1/4 cup/9
Roll	1/152
Mayonnaise	1 tbsp/100
Grapes	1/2 cup/30
Vegetable juice	12 oz (355 ml)/68
Carrot sticks	1/2 cup/28
Ranch dressing	1 tbsp/60
Snack	
Fat-free vanilla yogurt	1 cup/206
Low-fat granola	2 oz (57 g)/220
Dinner	
Chicken breast	3 oz (90 g)/168
Salsa	1/4 cup/18
Cheddar cheese	1 oz (30 g)/114
Spanish rice	1 1/2 cups/324
Snack	
Apple	1/80

Table 12.6 Menu 3

Food	Portion/calories
Breakfast	
Grape-Nuts	2 oz (60 g)/204
Cheerios	2 oz (60 g)/207
Skim milk	8 oz (250 ml)/86
Orange	1/70
Lunch	
Wheat bread	2 slices/130
Tuna	2 oz (60 g)/73
Mayonnaise	1 tbsp/100
Celery (chopped)	1/4 cup/5
Lettuce	1/2 cup/3
Apple juice	6 oz (175 ml)/87
Snack	
Crackers	12/120
Peanut butter	2 tbsp/188
Dinner	
Salmon (grilled)	3 oz (90 g)/118
Tossed salad	1 cup/22
Olive oil	1 tbsp (15 ml)/119
Broccoli	1 cup/52
Dinner roll	1/107
Vanilla ice cream	1/2 cup/133
Snack	
Fat-free vanilla yogurt	1 cup/206
Apple	1/80

SUMMARY

Healthy eating is not the same thing as dieting. Dieting implies a significant reduction in calories for the purpose of losing weight, usually in a short time. Most weight-loss diets involve unnatural eating patterns and too few nutrients for optimal physical function. Because such diets deprive you of important nutritional elements, most people cannot maintain diets very long, and almost all dieters regain all the weight they have lost within one year after discontinuing the diet.

The eating pattern recommended in the United States Department of Agriculture MyPlate plan is heart healthy and nutritious and can easily become part of a lifestyle that leads to improved physical well-being. You should find that a sound eating program provides plenty of energy and essential nutrients for performing your strength training workouts. However, people over age 50 need relatively high levels of protein to maximize muscle development. Once you have established a sensible nutrition plan, consider increasing your protein consumption for better muscle development. Also, try to ingest approximately 25 grams of protein shortly after your strength workouts for enhanced tissue building and muscle remodeling. In addition to eating plenty of protein-rich foods (because muscle is about 25 percent protein), be sure to drink six to eight 8-ounce glasses of water daily and more on workout days (because muscle is about 75 percent water).

References

Almstedt HC, Canepa JA, Ramirez DA, Shoepe TC. 2011. Changes in bone mineral density in response to 24 weeks of resistance training in college-age men and women. *Strength and Conditioning Research* 25(4): 1098-1103.

American College of Sports Medicine. 2009. Position stand: Exercise and physical activity for older adults. *Medicine and Science in Sports and Exercise* 41:1510-1530.

Annesi J, Westcott W. 2004. Relationship of feeling states after exercise and total mood disturbance over 10 weeks in formerly sedentary women. *Perceptual and Motor Skills* 99:107-115.

Annesi J, Westcott W. 2007. Relations of physical self-concept and muscular strength with resistance exercise-induced feeling states in older women. *Perceptual and Motor Skills* 104:183-190.

Baechle TR, Earle RW. 2014. *Fitness weight training, 3rd ed.* Champaign, IL: Human Kinetics.

Baechle TR, Groves, B. 1992. *Weight training: steps to success.* Champaign, IL: Human Kinetics.

Bircan C, Karasel SA, Akgun B, et al. 2008. Effects of muscle strengthening versus aerobic exercise program in fibromyalgia. *Rheumatology International* 28:527-532.

Boyle JP. Projection of the year 2050 burden of diabetes in the US adult population: Dynamic modeling of incidence, mortality, and prediabetes prevalence. *Population Health Metrics* 2010: 8(1):29.

Braith R, Graves J, Pollock M, et al. 1989. Comparison of two versus three days per week of variable resistance training during 10 and 18 week programs. *International Journal of Sports Medicine* 10:450-454.

Broeder C, Burrhus K, Svanevik L, Wilmore J. 1992. The effects of either high-intensity resistance or endurance training on resting metabolic rate. *American Journal of Clinical Nutrition* 55:802-810.

Busse AL, Filo WJ, Magaldi RM, et al. 2008. Effects of resistance training exercise on cognitive performance in elderly individuals with memory impairment: Results of a controlled trial. *Einstein* 6:402-407.

Campbell WW, Crim MC, Young VR, Evans WJ. 1994. Increased energy requirements and changes in body composition with resistance training in older adults. *American Journal of Clinical Nutrition* 60(2):167-175.

Campbell W, Trappe T, Wolfe R, and Evans W. 2001. The recommended dietary allowance for protein may not be adequate for older people to maintain skeletal muscle. *Journals of Gerontology Series A: Biological Sciences and Medical Sciences* 56:M373-M380.

Cassilhas RC, Viana VAR, Grasmann V, et al. 2007. The impact of resistance exercise on the cognitive function of the elderly. *Medicine and Science in Sports and Exercise* 39: 1401-1407.

Castaneda C, Layne JE, Munez-Orians L, et al. 2002. A randomized controlled trial of resistance exercise training to improve glycemic control in older adults with type 2 diabetes. *Diabetes Care* 25(12): 2335-2341.

Castro MJ, McCann DJ, Shaffrath JD, Adams WC. 1995. Peak torque per unit cross-sectional area differs between strength-trained and untrained young adults. *Medicine and Science In Sports and Exercise* 27(3):397-403.

DeMichele P, Pollock M, Graves J, et al. 1997. Isometric torso rotation strength: Effect of training frequency on its development. *Archives of Physical Medicine and Rehabilitation* 78:64-69.

Draovitch P, Westcott W. 1999. *Complete conditioning for golf.* Champaign, IL: Human Kinetics.

Dunstan DW, Daly RM, Owen N, et al. 2002. High-intensity resistance training improves glycemic control in older patients with type 2 diabetes. *Diabetes Care* 25(10):1729-1736.

Faigenbaum A, Skrinar G, Cesare W, et al. 1990. Physiologic and symptomatic responses of cardiac patients to resistance exercise. *Archives of Physical Medicine and Rehabilitation* 70:395-398.

Fiatarone MA, Marks E, Ryan N, et al. 1990. High-intensity strength training in nonagenarians. *Journal of the American Medical Association* 263(22):3029-3034.

Flack KD, Davy KP, Huber MAW, et al. 2011. Aging, resistance training, and diabetes prevention. *Journal of Aging Research* doi:10.4061/2011/127315.

Flegal KM, Carroll MD, Ogden CL, et al. 2010. Prevalence and trends in obesity among US adults, 1999-2008. *Journal of the American Medical Association* 303(3):235-241.

Focht BC. 2006. Effectiveness of exercise interventions in reducing pain symptoms among older adults with knee osteoarthritis: A review. *Journal of Aging and Physical Activity* 14:212-235.

Frontera WR, Hughes VA, Fiatarone MA, et al. 2000. Aging of skeletal muscle: A 12-yr longitudinal study. *Journal of Applied Physiology* 88:1321-1326.

Gutin B, Kasper MJ. 1992. Can exercise play a role in osteoporosis prevention? A review. *Osteoporosis International* 2:55-69.

Hackney KJ, Engels HJ, Gretebeck RJ. 2008. Resting energy expenditure and delayed-onset muscle soreness after full-body resistance training with an eccentric concentration. *Strength and Conditioning Research* 22(5):1602-1609.

Hayden JA, van Tulder MW, Tomlinson G. 2005. Systematic review: Strategies for using exercise therapy to improve outcomes in chronic low back pain. *Annals of Internal Medicine* 142:776-785.

Heden T, Lox C, Rose P, et al. 2011. One-set resistance training elevates energy expenditure for 72 hours similar to three sets. *European Journal of Applied Physiology* 111:477-484.

Hedley AA, Ogden CL, Johnson CL, et al. 2004. Obesity among U.S. children, adolescents, and adults, 1999-2002. *Journal of the American Medical Association* 291:2847-2850.

Holten MK, Zacho M, Gaster C, et al. 2004. Strength training increases insulin-mediated glucose uptake, GLUT4 content, and insulin signaling in skeletal muscle in patients with type 2 diabetes. *Diabetes* 53(2):294-305.

Johnston RE, Quinn TJ, Kertzer R, et al. 1995. Improving running economy through strength training. *Strength and Conditioning* 17(4):7-13.

Jones A, Pollock M, Graves J, et al. 1988. *Safe specific testing and rehabilitative exercise for the muscles of the lumbar spine.* Santa Barbara, CA: Sequoia Communications.

Katsanos CS, Kobayashi H, Sheffield-Moore M, et al. 2005. Aging is associated with diminished accretion of muscle proteins after the ingestion of a small bolus of essential amino acids. *American Journal of Clinical Nutrition* 82:165-73.

Keys A, Taylor HL, Grande F. 1973. Basal metabolism and age of adult man. *Metabolism* 22:579-587.

Kreuger J. 2004. Trends in strength training. *National Center for Chronic Disease and Health Promotion.*

Lange A, Vanwanseele B, Fiatarone Singh M. 2008. Strength training for treatment of osteoarthritis of the knee: A systematic review. *Arthritis and Rheumatology* 59:1488-1494.

Liddle SD, Baxter GD, Gracey JI. 2004. Exercise and chronic low back pain: What works? *Pain* 107:176-190.

Lloyd-Jones D, Adams R, Carnethon M, et al. 2009. Heart disease and stroke statistics: 2009 update. A report from the American Heart Association Statistics Committee and Stroke Statistics Subcommittee. *Circulation* 119:480-486.

Mann T, Tomiyama A, Westling E, et al. 2007. Medicare's search for effective obesity treatment; diets are not the answer. *American Psychologist* 62(3):220-233.

Marzolini S, Oh P, Thomas S, Goodman J. 2008. Aerobic and resistance training in coronary disease: Single versus multiple sets. *Medicine and Science in Sports and Exercise* 40:1557-1564.

Melov S, Tarnopolsky M, Beckman K, et al. 2007. Resistance exercise reverses aging in human skeletal muscle. *PLoS ONE* 2:e465.

National Osteoporosis Foundation. November 23 2009. Fast Facts. www.nof.org/osteoporosis/diseasefacts.htm.

Nelson ME, Fiatarone M, Morganti C., et al. 1994. Effects of high-intensity strength training on multiple risk factors for osteoporotic fractures. *Journal of the American Medical Association* 272: 1909-1914.

Ong KL, Cheung BMY, Man YB, et al. 2007. Hypertension treatment and control: Prevalence, awareness, treatment, and control of hypertension among United States adults 1999-2004. *Hypertension* 49:69-75.

Phillips SM, Winett RA. 2010. Uncomplicated resistance training and health-related outcomes: Evidence for a public health mandate. *Current Sports Medicine Reports* 9(4):208-213.

Pratley R, Nicklas B, Rubin M, et al. 1994. Strength training increases resting metabolic rate and norepinephrine levels in healthy 50- to 65-year-old men. *Journal of Applied Physiology* 76(1):133-137.

Risch S, Norvell N, Polock M, et al. 1993. Lumbar strengthening in chronic low back pain patients. *Spine* 18:232-238.

Schardt D. 2007. Saving muscle: How to stay strong and healthy as you age. *Nutrition Action Health Letter* 34(3):3-8.

Singh NA, Clements KM, Fiatarone MA. 1997. A randomized controlled trial of progressive resistance exercise in depressed elders. *Journal of Gerontology Series A: Biological Sciences and Medical Sciences* 52:M27-M35.

Standards of medical care in diabetes. 2006. *Diabetes Care* 29(1):S4-S42.

Starkey D, Pollock M, Ishida Y, et al. 1996. Effects of resistance training volume on strength and muscle thickness. *Medicine and Science in Sports and Exercise* 28(10): 1311-1320.

Stewart K, Mason M, Kelemen M. 1988. Three-year participation in circuit weight training improves muscular strength and self-efficacy in cardiac patients. *Journal of Cardiopulmonary Rehabilitation* 8:292-296.

Treuth MS, Ryan AS, Pratley RE, et al. 1994. Effects of strength training on total and regional body composition in older men. *Journal of Applied Physiology* 77(2):614-620.

Treuth MS, Hunter GR, Kekes-Szabo T, et al. 1995. Reduction in intra-abdominal adipose tissue after strength training in older women. *Journal of Applied Physiology* 78(4):1425-1431.

U.S. Department of Health and Human Services. 2004. *Bone Health and Osteoporosis: A Report of the Surgeon General.* Rockville, MD. U.S. Department of Health and Human Services, Public Health Service, Office of the Surgeon General.

Westcott WL. 1987. *Building strength at the YMCA.* Champaign, IL: Human Kinetics.

Westcott WL. 1994a. Weight loads: go figure. *Nautilus* 3(3)5-8.

Westcott WL. 1994b. Exercise speed and strength development. *American Fitness Quarterly* 3(3):20-21.

Westcott WL. 1995. Strength training for better running. *American Fitness Quarterly* 14(2):19-22.

Westcott WL. 2002. A new look at repetition ranges. *Fitness Management FMY* 18(8):36-37.

Westcott WL. 2009. Strength training for frail older adults. *Journal on Active Aging* 8(4):52-59.

Westcott WL. 2012. Resistance training is medicine: effects of strength training on health. *Current Sports Medicine Reports* 11(4):209-216.

Westcott WL, Apovian CM, Puhala K, et al. 2013. Nutrition programs enhance exercise effects on body composition and resting blood pressure. *Physician and Sportsmedicine* 41(3)85-91.

Westcott WL, Dolan F, Cavicchi T. 1996. Golf and strength training are compatible activities. *Strength and Conditioning* 18(4):54-56.

Westcott WL, Greenberger K, Milius D. 1989. Strength-training research: sets & repetitions. *Scholastic Coach* 58:98-100.

Westcott WL, Guy J. 1996. A physical evolution: Sedentary adults see marked improvements in as little as two days a week. *IDEA Today* 14(9):58-65.

Westcott WL, LaRosa Loud R. 1999. Strength, stretch, stamina. *Fitness Management* 15(6):44-45.

Westcott WL, LaRosa Loud R. 2013. Enhancing resistance training results with protein/carbohydrate supplementation. *ACSM's Health & Fitness Journal* 17(2):10-15.

Westcott WL, Parziale JR. 1997. Golf power. *Fitness Management* 13(13):39-41.

Westcott W, Varghese J, DiNubile N, et al. 2011. Exercise and nutrition more effective than exercise alone for increasing lean weight and reducing resting blood pressure. *Journal of Exercise Physiology* 14(4):120-133.

Westcott WL, Winett RA, Annesi JJ, et al. 2009. Prescribing physical activity: Applying the ACSM protocols for exercise type, intensity, and duration across 3 training frequencies. *Physician and Sportsmedicine* 2:51-58.

Wolfe RR. 2006. The unappreciated role of muscle in health and disease. *American Journal of Clinical Nutrition* 84:475-482.

About the Authors

Wayne L. Westcott, PhD, directs the exercise science program and fitness research program at Quincy College in Quincy, Massachusetts. He has been a strength training advisor for several national organizations, including the American Council on Exercise, American Senior Fitness Association, YMCA of the USA, President's Council on Physical Fitness and Sports, International Council on Active Aging, Medical Fitness Association, and United States Navy. He has also served as an editorial advisor for publications such as *Physician and Sports Medicine, American College of Sports Medicine's Health and Fitness Journal, American College of Sports Medicine's Certified News, Fitness Management, On-Site Fitness, American Fitness Quarterly, Club Industry, Perspective, Prevention, Men's Health,* and *Shape.*

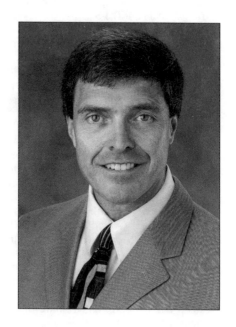

Westcott is the author of 25 fitness books, including *Building Strength and Stamina, Strength Training for Seniors, Fitness Professional's Guide to Strength Training Older Adults, Strength and Power for Young Athletes, Complete Conditioning for Golf, Youth Strength Training,* and *Building Strength and Stamina Navy Fitness Edition,* all with Human Kinetics.

Dr. Westcott has been honored with the Lifetime Achievement Award from the International Association of Fitness Professionals, the Healthy American Fitness Leader Award from the President's Council on Physical Fitness and Sports, the Roberts-Gulick Award from the YMCA Association of Professional Directors, the Lifetime Achievement Award from the Governor's Committee on Physical Fitness and Sports, the NOVA 7 Exercise Program Award from *Fitness Management Magazine,* the Marla Richmond Memorial Education Award from the Medical Fitness Association, the Alumni Recognition Award form the Pennsylvania State University, and the Faculty of the Year Award from Quincy College.

Thomas R. Baechle, EdD, CSCS,*D (R), NSCA-CPT,*D (R), is a professor and chair of the department of exercise science and pre health professions at Creighton University. He is a cofounder and past president of the National Strength and Conditioning Association (NSCA), and for 20 years he was the executive director of the NSCA Certification Commission.

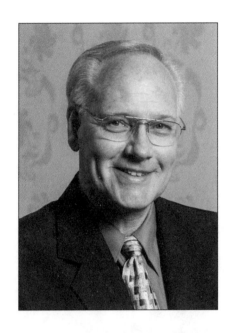

Baechle has received numerous awards, including the Lifetime Achievement Award from the NSCA and the Excellence in Teaching Award from Creighton University. He has more than 35 years of experience competing in and coaching weightlifting and powerlifting and presenting and teaching on these topics. Baechle has authored, coauthored, or edited 16 books, including three editions of *Fitness Weight Training,* four editions of the popular *Weight Training: Steps to Success,* one edition of the accompanying instructor guide, one edition of *Essentials of Personal Training,* and three editions of *Essentials of Strength Training and Conditioning,* all published by Human Kinetics, some of which have been translated into more than 10 languages.

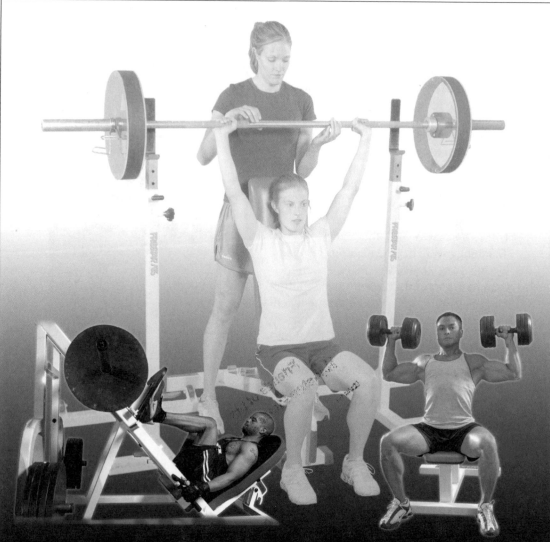

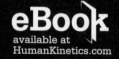